Seven Steps to

Nighttime Dryness

A Practical Guide for Parents
of Children with Bedwetting

By Renee Mercer
Certified Pediatric Nurse Practitioner

Brookeville Media   Ashton, Maryland

First printing 2004.

Visit www.bedwettinghandbook.com for additional bedwetting information and resources mentioned in this book.

Publication Date: January, 2004

Brookeville Media LLC
PO Box 27
Ashton, MD 20861
www.brookevillemedia.com

ISBN 0-9740688-0-2

LCCN 2003111357

Attention Corporations, Universities, Colleges, and Professional Organizations:
Quantity discounts are available on bulk purchases of this book for educational, gift purposes, or as premiums. For information, please contact Brookeville Media LLC, PO Box 27, Ashton, MD 20861. 301-774-9835.

Subject area: Parenting/Childcare

Book design: EnZed Design, Denver
Cover illustration: Linda Bronson, Getty Images
Edited by: Lynn Gorham Johnson

About the Author

Renee Mercer is a Certified Pediatric Nurse Practitioner specializing in the treatment of children with enuresis, or bedwetting. She sees children with bedwetting and daytime wetting in her private practice, Enuresis Associates, in Ellicott City, Maryland. Renee has more than 20 years of experience in pediatrics. She developed her interest in enuresis after appreciating the great unmet need of children with bedwetting. She works closely with families in their quest for dryness and has a tremendous success rate.

After years of frustration finding suitable products for children with bedwetting, Renee co-founded the Bedwetting Store, (www.bedwetting store.com) a comprehensive online and catalog source for bedwetting alarms, waterproof bedding and pads, products for daytime wetting and information to assist children in achieving dryness.

Renee lives with her husband and three sons in Maryland.

CONTENTS

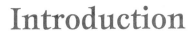

Introduction

When a child stays dry during the day, yet still wets at night, everyone involved becomes frustrated. Parents often wonder if they are doing something to keep their child from staying dry at night. They may feel embarrassed that their 6-year-old (or 10-year-old, or teenager) is wetting the bed; the child is probably embarrassed, too. Parents may wonder if their child is simply lazy (or even bad). Most of all, they wonder about what they can do to help their child stop wetting the bed.

For more than 20 years, I have been a pediatric nurse practitioner and developed a special interest in the medical condition called enuresis, or bedwetting. I have a private practice, Enuresis Associates, in Ellicott City, Maryland, through which I've helped hundreds of children learn to stay dry around the clock. I developed my interest in enuresis after finding that, despite the fact that about five million school-age children in the United States wet the bed, very few resources exist for them in this country. As a result, I developed my practice, as well as a catalog and online bedwetting resource store. Every day, I see frustration, embarrassment and helplessness on the faces of the children and parents I help. Together, using simple techniques, we solve their children's bedwetting and end the negative emotions they may feel.

During my years of practice, I have learned many practical tips from my patients and developed useful techniques that work. I understand that each child and his family situation is unique. Also, I know that most parents are very loving and want to do "what's best" for their bedwetting child, but many have no idea where and when to begin. This book will not only give you a starting point, but easy-to-follow steps leading to dry nights.

Families whose children have never had a night of bedwetting might congratulate themselves and rejoice in what good parents they are, offering no support for families with bedwetting. Please be assured that bedwetting is not due to a parent deficit, any more than diabetes or attention deficit disorders are. Children with bedwetting are not lazy. They are great students, athletes, musicians and generally wonderful kids.

Many things can cause bedwetting, including heredity, decreased sleep arousal and large nighttime urine production, just to name a few. No two children are alike, and a factor that may play a large role in one child's bedwetting may have little to do with the bedwetting of another.

Children with bedwetting all go to bed hoping that tonight will be the night they wake up dry. After reading this book, you will understand the steps to take that will help your child fulfill this hope. I offer no magic solution, but rather these practical tips and knowledge to assist you in the quest for dryness.

I want to emphasize that you do not have to "wait for your child to grow out of it," as is suggested by many well-meaning health-care providers and relatives. It is true that less than 1 percent of 18-year-olds wet the bed, so maturation does play a role. However, treating a 6-year-old who has nightly bedwetting is easier than a 13-year-old. And bedwetting has not impacted the 6-year-old's social life as greatly. Being wet at night can become a distant childhood memory, regardless of a child's age. By treating bedwetting now, the amount of time that it takes for a child to stop wetting independently can often be decreased by many years.

How to use this book

As the title says, this book breaks down the process of helping your child stay dry at night into seven steps. Using this logical progression, you will eliminate other ineffective treatments and have concrete knowledge that you are on the right track. I encourage you to read the steps in order; jumping ahead may cause you to miss a point that could be key to your child's success. Here is a brief overview of what you can expect to learn in each step:

- **Step 1: Review the basics.** You'll learn how the urinary system works, what causes bedwetting and what myths may be coloring your approach to solving the problem.
- **Step 2: Select the right time to start.** You'll learn how to assess when both you and your child are ready to tackle this issue; if both of you aren't ready, you will sabotage effective treatment.
- **Step 3: Pick the right treatment for your child.** You'll learn about the different treatments available and formulate your action plan.
- **Step 4: Choose a bedwetting alarm.** You'll learn about this crucial treatment tool and how to determine which type is right for your child's specific needs.
- **Step 5: Prepare to use your bedwetting alarm.** You'll learn the essential things to do to get yourself, your child and his environment ready for using an alarm.
- **Step 6: Use your alarm until your child is consistently dry.** You'll learn what to expect from your child and how to handle setbacks along the way.
- **Step 7: Know when to stop.** You'll learn how to determine when to stop treatment to ensure your child's new behavior is permanent.

Look to page 81 for some of the common questions and answers I've been presented with over the years. Perhaps you will see your own family situation in some of them. Remember, each child is different, and their responses are different, but these techniques do work! By following my seven steps, most children will achieve dry nights. Imagine no more declined sleepover invitations or increased laundry chores. Your child will be sleeping comfortably and dry. Good luck!

Part 1:
The Seven Steps

Review the basics

Bedwetting defined

Bedwetting is defined as the nightly release of urine by children older than 6 who should have developed nighttime dryness. It is also known as *nocturnal enuresis*. About 90 percent of children who wet the bed have *always* wet the bed; they are considered to have *primary enuresis*. The other 10 percent or so have experienced at least six months of dryness, then resume wetting, a condition called *secondary enuresis*. For the purposes of this book, we will talk mostly about *primary nocturnal enuresis*.

The urinary system

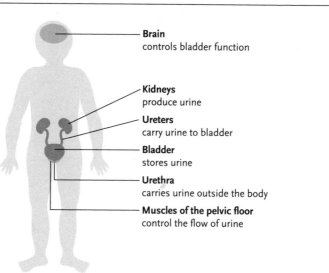

Brain
controls bladder function

Kidneys
produce urine

Ureters
carry urine to bladder

Bladder
stores urine

Urethra
carries urine outside the body

Muscles of the pelvic floor
control the flow of urine

How the urinary system works

Before you begin to understand bedwetting, it may be helpful to understand how the urinary system works. The urinary system is responsible for producing urine (one of the body's waste products), storing it and getting rid of it. The system is comprised of six parts.

David's Story

David is 7 and wets his bed every night. His father remembers bedwetting. His mother is concerned because she allows him to wear disposable pants at night. David's parents wonder what exactly causes bedwetting and what, if anything, they are doing to contribute to it.

- **Kidneys.** A paired organ located in your mid to lower back that produces urine.
- **Ureters.** Tubes that carry urine from your kidneys to your storage unit, the bladder.
- **Bladder.** A small, muscular balloon that is your body's urine storage unit. Your bladder's walls relax to fill with urine and contract to squeeze it out. Everyone's bladder capacity is different—ranging from about eight to 14 ounces (1 to 1¾ cups) of urine.
- **Urethra.** The tube that carries urine from your bladder to outside your body. Girls have a short urethra and boys have a longer one. Your urethra passes through the pelvic floor muscles.
- **Pelvic floor muscles.** These muscles, located in your groin, help control the flow of urine. By consciously squeezing these muscles, you can stop the flow of urine until you find a toilet. (You might know them as your Kegel muscles.)
- **Brain.** Your brain controls much of this operation, just as it does other body systems. When your bladder reaches its full capacity, it sends messages to your brain through your nervous system to let you know you need to use the toilet. If your brain doesn't receive these messages, or if it doesn't know how to make you respond properly to the message, wetting can occur.

The urinary system of most children with bedwetting works just fine. The problem may lie more in how their brains and bladders coordinate the messages and, especially, in how your child responds to those messages in the middle of the night.

To put bedwetting into perspective, recognize that children develop urinary control as they mature. Everyone is born wetting day and night. As a child grows and develops, so does his ability to control his bladder.

Between ages 1 and 2, his bladder capacity will gradually enlarge and he will begin to sense when his bladder is full. At ages 3 to 4, he learns to voluntarily void or inhibit voiding. By age 5, a typical child has an adult pattern of urinary control. However, approximately 13 percent of 6-year-olds don't yet have nighttime urinary control and still have bed-wetting episodes.[1]

How common is bedwetting?

Nocturnal enuresis is common among children throughout the world. In the United States, bedwetting affects an estimated five to seven million children over age 5—a significant percentage of school-aged children. At age 10, one in 20 children have bedwetting. By age 15, 1 to 6 percent wet the bed.

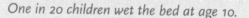

One in 20 children wet the bed at age 10.

Estimated prevalence of nocturnal enuresis in children

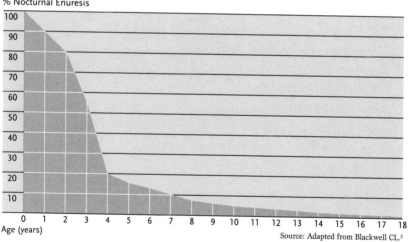

Source: Adapted from Blackwell CL.[2]

Bedwetting can be inherited

Many parents of bedwetters were bedwetters themselves. Researchers have documented a greater incidence of bedwetting in children whose parents were bedwetters when compared to families with no parental history.[3] In fact, scientists have identified a "bedwetting gene," and the incidence of bedwetting increases if one or both parents wet the bed.[4]

Chance of enuresis in a child with positive family history

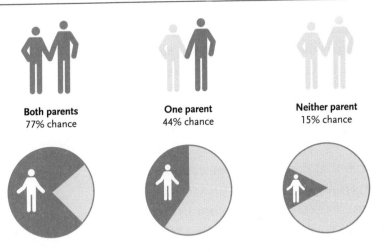

Both parents	One parent	Neither parent
77% chance	44% chance	15% chance

- In most studies, the father was more often affected than the mother, which is consistent with the fact that bedwetting is more common in boys than girls. The ratio of boys to girls has been reported to be 1.5 to 1.
- Research indicates that children are likely to stop bedwetting on their own at about the same age as the affected parent.[5] If the parent's bedwetting did not end until the teen years, successful intervention in a 6-year-old will decrease the total wet time by years.
- Positive family history is not limited to parents. Uncles, aunts or grandparents may have been similarly affected but reluctant to share this information. When questioned, they may remember wet nights as a child. Sharing these bits of information with your child will help him realize that wetting the bed is not his fault; it is an inherited trait.

Like many parents, you may have distinct memories of situations you endured because of your own bedwetting. Effective bedwetting treatment and specially designed products did not exist 30 years ago. People at that time viewed bedwetting as a psychological problem. Some families chose to punish, ridicule and embarrass the bedwetting child as a means of stopping the problem. These techniques rarely decreased the number of wet nights and certainly damaged the child's self esteem.

If you are a parent who wet the bed as a child, you may have endured punishment for something you could not control. You made it to adulthood despite this misguided approach; however, you certainly should not punish your own child for bedwetting. Today, we know much more about enuresis. Although we cannot pinpoint a single causative factor, we do know that children do not wet on purpose, and in most cases, psychological disturbances don't cause bedwetting.

Factors that don't cause bedwetting

Poor parenting

Because bedwetting can be inherited, it's common for more than one child in a family to be affected. Sometimes, every child in a family wets at night. It is difficult for parents not to blame themselves or feel inadequate because bedwetting affects *their* children and not those of their relatives or friends. Your child does not wet the bed because you are a poor parent. However, good parenting—being accepting, supportive and not punitive—can help your child stop bedwetting.

Supporting your child is crucial to success.

Lazy children

Parents report that they think their bedwetting child is just lazy—he doesn't *want* to get out of bed to go to the bathroom, so he lays there and urinates. Common sense says no child really wants to wake up in a wet bed. Every child will choose dryness, if only he has that choice. A child will rarely wet the bed on purpose.

Children with bedwetting are not lazy! They are good kids who feel they have no control over their bedwetting. They feel frustrated, too. They all go to bed hoping that this will be the night they wake up dry.

Factors that cause bedwetting

The newest information indicates that bedwetting is caused by many factors.[6] Because we know no single, simple cause, we have no single, simple cure. Some factors that play a role in bedwetting are:

- Decreased arousal from sleep in response to a full bladder
- Small functional bladder capacity
- High nighttime urine production
- Food sensitivities
- Constipation
- Other factors

Key factors in enuresis

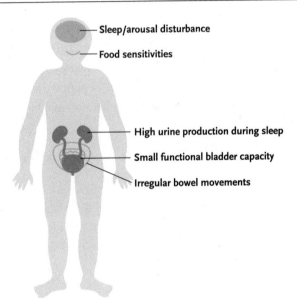

- Sleep/arousal disturbance
- Food sensitivities
- High urine production during sleep
- Small functional bladder capacity
- Irregular bowel movements

We'll investigate each factor in detail below.

Decreased arousal from sleep

No parent whose child wets at night will tell you the child is a light sleeper (easily aroused). Bedwetting is not caused by deep sleep, and it is not a true sleep disorder. But for reasons we don't quite understand, it seems that children with bedwetting do not spontaneously wake up when their bladders are full.[7] They have a decreased sleep arousal phenomenon; we think their arousal system is slow to mature. Children in general are less likely than adults to arouse from deep sleep because adults' arousal system is fully developed.

Bedwetting can occur at all stages and levels of sleep. If the child has decreased arousal from sleep, his brain and bladder aren't able to communicate about what to do when his bladder is full. He doesn't wake up to urinate in the toilet. Instead, his muscles relax, allowing his bladder to empty while he sleeps.

Small functional bladder capacity

Your child's functional bladder capacity is the point at which his brain receives his bladder's message that it is full and needs to empty. Small bladder capacity may play a part in bedwetting. To determine your child's bladder capacity, you'll need a measuring container. Have your child urinate into the container about 10 separate times over three days. The largest recorded measurement is his functional bladder capacity. A good rule of thumb:

$$\textbf{child's age} + \textbf{2} = \textbf{ounces of average bladder capacity}[8]$$

For example, an 11-year-old should be able to hold 13 ounces of urine at a time without difficulty. It is not unusual for a bedwetting child's bladder capacity to be much smaller than average for his age. Children who wet commonly have both decreased arousal from sleep and a small functional bladder capacity.

Continued urine production

Under normal circumstances, urine production is controlled by a substance known as anti-diuretic hormone (ADH). At night, the brain increases release of ADH, causing a smaller amount of urine to be produced. That's why you don't have to get up to urinate every few hours at night like you do during the day. Some children with bedwetting don't seem to produce more ADH at bedtime.[9] If a child's ADH doesn't rise at night, his kidneys continue to produce dilute urine in daytime amounts.

Children who are easily aroused from sleep simply wake up at night to eliminate this larger amount of urine. But children with decreased sleep arousal don't feel the urge to wake up and urinate in the bathroom. They sleep through urinating in their beds.

Food sensitivities

Food sensitivities may contribute to enuresis. Having a food sensitivity doesn't mean a child is "allergic" to that particular food, but that the food may affect their urinary system or sleep system. Each person's response to certain foods is unique. For example, drinking a carbonated beverage in the evening may cause a "flood" in one child and have absolutely no effect on another.

If you know the effects certain foods and drinks have on your child's body, you can control the amount of urine your child produces. For example, tea has a well-known diuretic effect. Many people notice they urinate more often and in larger quantities after drinking tea than if they had the same amount of another fluid. Again, each response is individual. In children with bedwetting, what they drink may increase their urine production and thus increase wetting episodes. By identifying the offending foods or fluids, your child can make wise choices.

Some researchers suggest that foods and substances such as milk and milk products, caffeine, Vitamin C and citrus juices, heavily sugared foods and carbonated beverages may contribute to enuresis.[10] To determine if your child is sensitive to these foods, you'll need to conduct a "food challenge." Eliminate these trigger foods from his diet for two weeks, and then gradually reintroduce them one at a time, every three to four days. On particularly wet nights, note what new food was added, remove it from your child's diet again, then "challenge" him with the same food a few days later. If your child consistently wets the bed when he ingests this food, encourage him to eliminate it from his diet, especially when staying dry is of the utmost importance. For example, if lemonade causes daytime urgency or bedwetting, and a sleepover is coming up, suggest that he drink other beverages that night to help maintain dryness.

Foods that may contribute to wetting

- Carbonated drinks
- Artificial colors
- Citric acid (oranges, lemons)
- Milk and dairy, especially after lunchtime
- Sugary foods and candy
- Vitamin supplements, especially Vitamin C
- Caffeinated beverages, chocolate

If your child is a sound sleeper, you might pay particular attention to whether he is consuming milk and dairy products in the evening. These foods contain tryptophan, an amino acid that triggers serotonin release. Serotonin in turn allows you to sleep more soundly. There is no need to further compromise a sound sleeper's decreased sleep arousal!

Constipation

Constipation and infrequent stools can play a role in enuresis. One theory is that a full rectum restricts the bladder's expansion and causes the bladder to contract even though it isn't full. Another theory is that a full rectum's constant rubbing of the bladder decreases the bladder's sensitivity and causes the brain to begin ignoring messages from that area.[10] Many school-age children with bedwetting have infrequent, firm stools. Parents are often unaware of this, so it is necessary to gather this information from your child. Simply increasing dietary fiber is often enough to ensure a soft stool every one to two days. High-fiber cereal is a tasty way to get a few additional grams of fiber into your child's diet each day.

Other factors

School schedules can impact thirst and, ultimately, bedwetting. Often, short lunch periods keep kids from finishing their mealtime drink. Children need access to a water bottle or drinking fountain, as well as time to finish their lunchtime beverage, to stay hydrated. If they don't have enough to drink during the school day, they will come home very thirsty. Instead of spreading their total daily fluid intake over 12 hours, they crunch it into the late afternoon and evening. Their bodies then excrete the waste during the night.

Another issue: the school bathroom. Many school-aged children are reluctant to use the school bathroom, or they do not have enough time between classes to go. Remind your child that it is healthy for his bladder and bowel to empty on a regular basis. Provide a note to his teacher if this is a source of frustration for him.

Medications that children take may influence bedwetting. Certain anti-depressant medications cause increased thirst and increased urine production, which may cause secondary enuresis. Anti-psychotic/anti-anxiety medications may change your child's sleep pattern or increase relaxation of muscles that control urination. Antihistamines, allergy medications and cold-and-cough preparations taken at bedtime may make your child sleep more soundly, and thus not wake up to use the toilet on nights he takes the medication. Sometimes changing your child's dosing pattern to earlier in the day will decrease the effect on nighttime wetting. Always consult with your health-care provider before changing any medication schedules.

Children with *attention or learning problems* have a higher incidence of bedwetting than children in the general population.[11] The reason is not clear. Many families find when the attention problem is addressed and under control, bedwetting decreases or the child responds more readily to treatment. It is important to note that bedwetting may be a common problem for children with learning disabilities, but bedwetting *alone* does not *predict* learning disabilities. In other words, the fact that a child wets the bed does not mean he has learning problems.

Secondary nocturnal enuresis, in which the child has resumed wetting after at least six consecutive months of dryness, can have even more causes. Infections, diabetes, eating disorders, encopresis (severe constipation) and emotional upheaval should be ruled out. Bedwetting after a long period of dryness should be brought to your health-care provider's attention. A few simple medical tests can ensure your child has no new physical reasons for restarting the wetting. Unfortunately, it's common not to find the exact cause of bedwetting resurgence. If the wetting persists after mental and physical reasons for enuresis have been treated, children will often respond to the same treatments as children with primary nocturnal enuresis.

Urinary problems are rare in children with primary bedwetting, but your health-care provider should consider them. Such problems include urinary tract infections, spinal cord abnormalities, irritable bladders, posterior urethral valves in boys or ectopic ureter in girls. Only three in 100 bedwetting children have a physical abnormality that causes the bedwetting. The rest have normal urinary systems. If your child has had urinary tract infections or has problems with daytime wetting, the likelihood that there is a physical problem increases.

Ten common myths and facts about bedwetting

1. You have to wait for your child to outgrow bedwetting.

Although 15 percent of bedwetting children stop wetting on their own each year, that means 85 percent will still be wetting this time next year.[12] Because we now have safe, effective techniques to help your child eliminate bedwetting, there is no reason that you have to wait for years for bedwetting to stop spontaneously. When your family has become frustrated with laundry and begins making excuses for sleepovers, it is time for intervention. Your child should be around 6 before you start.

2. Most children with bedwetting have mental or physical problems.

Only three in 100 children with primary nocturnal enuresis have a physical or urologic cause for it. Psychological problems as a cause of primary bedwetting are not common. Even children with emotional challenges can respond to treatment for bedwetting.

3. If a child is a sound sleeper, a bedwetting alarm won't work for her.

It is true that children with bedwetting may have a higher threshold for loud noise than other children. Initially the alarm is for the parents—so they can help wake the child and accompany her to the bathroom. Over time, the child begins to associate the noise with stopping the flow of urine and going to the toilet. Gradually, she will learn to control her muscles in response to a full bladder instead of relaxing them as she has done in the past.

Seven Steps to Nighttime Dryness

4. If the child doesn't tell her parents she is bothered by her bedwetting, she probably doesn't care if she is wet.

No child wants to wake up in a wet bed. As children reach school age and realize their peers don't wear disposable pants or worry about waking to a wet bed, their self-esteem and social independence are affected. By middle school, their age-appropriate activities are sharply curtailed. All children would rather be dry, and if given ways to control this, are very cooperative with treatments and the use of bedwetting alarms.

5. Bedwetting is nothing more than a pesky problem that will eventually go away.

Perhaps, but with effective treatment available, why wait until your child outgrows it? Financially, enuresis impacts families. One or two extra loads of laundry each day can cost as much as $700 each year. Disposable pants can easily add up to $300 a year. Medications for bedwetting can cost $4 per tablet, and even $25 prescription drug copays add up over time.

Emotionally, enuresis impacts families. Overnight arrangements are cumbersome—taking along waterproof sheets, disposable pants, extra clothing, etc. Hiding enuresis from other family members and friends is painful. Peers and siblings can be cruel, teasing or humiliating the affected child. Parents must make every effort to prevent teasing from siblings. Remind siblings that they may have challenges in certain aspects of their lives, too. Bedwetting is not done on purpose. Your family works together to overcome challenges.

6. My child is alone in having this problem.

If a parent, grandparent, aunt or uncle with a history of bedwetting can share their memories with your child, it will help her see that she is not so different. Learning that an adult she respects and admires was similarly affected may help. Also remind your child that, in a class of 25 8-year-olds, at least one or two other children wet the bed.

7. Bedwetting occurred because I left him in disposable pants too long.

Most children are day toilet trained between ages 2 and 4. There are generally three types of children where it comes to nighttime dryness:

- Those who become spontaneously dry at night.
- Those who begin with an occasional dry night, progress to more dry nights than wet ones and achieve complete dryness without intervention, usually by 6. Parents of these children should assist them in removing their disposable pants immediately after wakening in the morning and urinating in the toilet. Disposable pants can be discontinued as dry nights prevail.
- Those who have had very few, if any, dry nights in their lives. These children may wet no matter where they are, how much their fluids are restricted or even if their parents take them to the toilet during the night. Using disposable pants in this group can decrease parent frustration until a treatment program is in place.

8. Parents should restrict privileges or punish their children so they will become dry quicker.
Remember, your child does not consciously control her bedwetting. Punishing your child for an activity that she has no control over is counterproductive. Dealing with the wetting in a supportive manner, such as having your child help make her bed or carry her bedding to and from the washer should be viewed as sharing in household tasks, not as punishment.

9. Puberty will end bedwetting.
It's true that the number of children with bedwetting decreases with age, but even 1 percent of 18-year-olds continue to have bedwetting. Puberty does not cure bedwetting, and there is no reason that you should wait until your child approaches this age before you attempt treatment.

10. Medication is a sure cure for bedwetting.
Although medications such as DDAVP *(desmopressin)* or Ditropan *(oxybutynin)* work well as an adjunct to therapy and in instances where a child has to be dry (camps or overnight visits), use of medication alone rarely helps a child permanently overcome bedwetting. When the medication is stopped, the wetting returns in 80 to 90 percent of those

treated. Medication can help to buy time in some families who are not ready to use a bedwetting alarm. Children who use alarms are nine times more likely to become dry and stay dry than those who use medication alone.[13]

References

1 Fergusson DM, Hons BA, Horwood LJ, et al. Factors related to the age of attainment of nocturnal bladder control: An 8-year longitudinal study. Pediatrics. 1986; 78:884-890.
2 Blackwell CL. A Guide to Enuresis. A Guide for Treatment of Enuresis for Professionals. United Kingdom. Enuresis Resource and Information Centre; 1995.
3 Arnell H et al. The genetics of primary nocturnal enuresis: Inheritance and suggestion of a second major gene on chromosome 12q. J Med Genet. 1997; 34: 360-365.
4 Eiberg H, Berendt I, Mohr J. Assignment of dominant inherited nocturnal enuresis (ENURI) to chromosome 13q. Nat Genet. 1985; 10: 354-356.
5 See Fergusson.
6 Mercer R. Dry at Night. Treating Nocturnal Enuresis. Adv Nurse Pract. 2003; 11:26-31.
7 Schmitt BD. Nocturnal Enuresis. Pediatr Rev. 1997; 18:183-190.
8 Maizels M, Rosenbaum D, Keating B. Getting to Dry: How to Help Your Child Overcome Bedwetting. Boston. The Harvard Common Press; 1999.
9 Rittig S et al. Abnormal diurnal rhythm of plasma vasopressin and urinary output in patients with enuresis. Am J Physiol. 1989. 363: 6127-6189.
10 See Maizels
11 Robson WL et al. Enuresis in children with attention-deficit hyperactivity disorder. South Med J. 1997; 90: 503-505.
12 See Schmitt
13 Bosson S, Lyth N. Nocturnal enuresis. In Barton S, ed. Clinical Evidence. Issue 5. London. BMJ Publishing; 2001; 6:300-305.

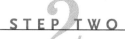
Select the right time to start

The best time to begin treating bedwetting is when it starts to become an issue. There is no consensus as to an absolute time for any child. The timing depends more on what is right for each family. When your child is about 6, makes comments about wanting to be dry, is still wearing disposable pants to bed, or notices that her younger sibling is dry, it may be a good time for intervention. Some children may not be concerned about bedwetting until they are 7 or 8 and are invited to sleep at a friend's house. Certainly, intervention should take place by age 8, but do not be disheartened if your child is 9 or older and you are just learning about bedwetting treatment. They, too, will get to dryness, but it may take longer with older children.

Factors in choosing when to start treatment

Deciding when your family and your child are both ready to work on achieving nighttime dryness is very individual. The following are things you should consider:

■ **Your child's temperament.** Some children naturally worry more than others. They worry that there is something wrong with them or that they are different from their peers. Other children are more easygoing and easily make accommodations for sleepovers. As a parent, you know your child's temperament better than anyone. Early intervention and much reassurance is helpful for the "worrier."

■ **Family stressors.** Taking these steps to dryness requires effort from both parents and child, so it's helpful to choose a low-stress time to begin. (As parents, you may laugh and ask, What is that?) High-stress times may be: immediately before holidays or family vacations; at the beginning of the school year; when your child is starting a new sport; following a sibling's birth; following a close family member's death; during or following a divorce; and while or following moving.

Stephanie is 9 and in third grade. Her best friend excitedly brought invitations to a birthday sleepover to school. Stephanie had tears in her eyes as she told her mother about the invitation. She told her friend she had other plans that night, although the real reason she couldn't attend was her bedwetting. Stephanie's parents have been very patient in waiting for her to "outgrow" her nightly wetting, but now they know they need to do something else.

When you have a fairly regular schedule, without a lot of added concerns, it's a good time to work on achieving dryness.

- **Your child's goals or obligations.** Your child might mention to you that she would really like to sleep at her friend's house without disposable pants or go to a week of camp with her friends next summer. These are often very realistic goals and indicate her level of motivation.

- **Your child's age.** Each child develops at a different rate, but the average child is dry at night by age 6. Some 5-year-olds are very motivated to become dry, whereas some 7-year-olds are not.

- **Whether they have had any dry nights.** In a 5- or 6-year-old who is having dry nights about half the time, supportive treatment may be all that is necessary as she continues to develop. However, a 6-year-old who has never had a dry night is less likely to get to dryness without intervention. In an older child, for example age 10 or 11, wetting even a few nights a week is too much. Intervention to get to complete dryness is warranted. Remind your child that there is help for bedwetting and a number of treatment options are available to make things better for her.

Talking to your child's health-care provider

About 97 percent of bedwetting children who are dry during the day have no medical problems that cause their bedwetting. For that reason, many health-care providers view bedwetting as a non-medical problem and, although well-meaning, they may not recommend any form of treatment. In fact, they may tell you to do nothing while you wait for your child to outgrow it. Because bedwetting is rarely caused by a medical problem, many physicians have no training in or knowledge of the most effective methods for resolving bedwetting.

That said, it is still important that you discuss the fact that your child is wetting the bed with your child's health-care provider. Her doctor will perform a thorough physical exam, including an external exam of her genitalia. Most children will have normal exams. During the exam, your child's doctor or nurse practitioner should also collect the following information:

- **Age of daytime dryness.** A developmentally delayed child may achieve nighttime dryness later than a typical child.
- **Urgency or frequency in the daytime.** Parents often describe this as "waiting too long, and having to run to the bathroom." Daytime frequency may indicate a small bladder capacity.
- **Daytime leaking.** Does leaking occur on the way to the bathroom or as "dribbling" in the underwear after they feel they have finished urinating? Does your child feel the urge to urinate or just look down and see wet underwear? Daytime leaking symptoms may be more indicative of urologic problems.
- **Infrequent stools or constipation.** A full bowel can further compromise the ability of the bladder to fully expand.
- **Adequacy of their urine stream.** Children should have a strong stream when emptying a full bladder.
- **History of urinary tract infections or other kidney problems.** Urinary tract and kidney problems may make achieving nighttime dryness more difficult.

Your provider may perform a urinalysis in the office to check for signs of infection, concentrating problems or sugar elevations. If your child's levels are normal, she usually won't require any further lab tests. If the results are abnormal or your doctor has other concerns, she may recommend other tests.

Some associated medical conditions make treating bedwetting more difficult. Although these occur in only a tiny percentage of children, I have described them below:

- Urinary symptoms such as daytime leaking and wetting should be treated before addressing nighttime dryness. Frequent or recent urinary tract infections (UTIs) may indicate a urologic problem that should be ruled out as a cause for bedwetting.

■ Constipation may interfere with your child's ability to become dry at night. Having a regular, soft stool in the toilet every day or two is important. If this is a problem for your child, you might begin with increasing her daily fiber intake and bringing it to her doctor's attention.

■ Diabetes mellitus, because of increased thirst and increased urine production, can present with bedwetting. Your doctor or nurse practitioner can do a urine test to make sure diabetes mellitus isn't a contributing factor. In some children, bedwetting was present before the diabetes. Once their diabetes is under control, these children can learn to wake up and go to the bathroom to urinate.

■ Another type of diabetes, diabetes insipidus, is a condition in which the body cannot concentrate the urine and always produces a profuse amount of very dilute urine. Your child can be screened for this on a routine urine test. If your doctor suspects this is a problem, more extensive tests and medication may be necessary.

■ Sleep apnea, a rare condition in which your child stops breathing for a few seconds during sleep, can be associated with bedwetting. Obstructive tonsils, mouth breathing or snoring could alert you that sleep apnea might be a contributing factor. Sleep studies can determine if sleep apnea is present.

Secondary enuresis

Secondary enuresis is bedwetting that starts after at least six months of dryness. Medical or psychological causes are more common in children with secondary enuresis than in those with primary enuresis—those who have always wet the bed. Secondary enuresis may be triggered by:

■ Life changes such as parent's divorce, a death, a major move or a family upheaval

■ Recent illness, such as streptococcal or viral illness

■ Eating disorders, such as anorexia nervosa

■ Starting medications such as anti-depressants, anti-psychotics or allergy treatments

Children with secondary enuresis should see a doctor to rule out other conditions before starting bedwetting treatment. In some cases, we never pinpoint why a child resumed bedwetting. Whether the cause is determined and treated, or we never discover a cause, children who resume bedwetting will usually respond to the treatments discussed in this book.

Ending bedwetting improves self-esteem

Children with bedwetting may have lower self-esteem, but their self-concept improves when bedwetting is cured.[1] Children with enuresis often go to great lengths to hide their wetting from family members and friends. Parents report finding wet sheets and clothing while their child denies that she wets. These children often avoid sleepovers altogether or make excuses to be picked up early. As your child reaches middle and high school, she may avoid overnight school trips and camps. Enuresis can impact her normal development of independence. Shame, inferiority and feelings of isolation are common. Often your child feels she is the only one with this problem.

Treatment is beneficial. Research indicates that negative feelings dissipate once the bedwetting is cured. Children who have received treatment for nocturnal enuresis have improved scores in social behavior and self-concept. Emotional support and encouragement are important components of successful treatment for children with bedwetting.

References
[1] Longstaffe S, Moffatt M, Whalen J. Behavioral and self-concept changes after six months of enuresis treatment: A randomized, controlled trial. Pediatrics (Supp). 2000; 105: 935-940.

Pick the right treatment for your child

Curing bedwetting requires a sense of partnership regardless of the technique you choose. It's important to help your child view bedwetting as one of life's challenges. You can work together to solve this problem and give him a feeling of mastery over the situation. You can enlist his input in the type of treatment he would be most likely to use. Remind him that the things in life that you have worked the hardest for are also the ones that make you the most proud. Working hard to stay dry is something to be proud of!

Michael's Story

Michael is 9 and would love to attend a week of summer camp next year. Several of his friends have asked him if he will be going, but he doesn't know how to answer them. He and his parents have decided that they will work hard to curtail his bedwetting. They want to know what options they have to enable their son to go to camp with his friends next summer.

Before starting, consider this

A child struggling with enuresis may be somewhat consoled to know that Dad also wet until he was 10, as well as by the fact it is not his fault he has this problem. You can gauge how many more years your child will still wet without intervention by asking about the age at which a relative stopped bedwetting. Children often stop bedwetting at around the same time the relative did. In some cases, however, children continue wetting beyond the age of the affected relative. Intervention is particularly helpful in this group.

About 15 percent of children who wet the bed stop without intervention each year. While that's hopeful news, it also means 85 out of 100 children who wet will continue to do so this time next year if no intervention takes place. The majority of children with enuresis will need help to sleep dry and comfortably for a few years or will need assistance in stopping bedwetting permanently.

Treatment approaches

Treatment approaches generally fall into two categories: supportive and curative. *Supportive* interventions help "buy time" until your child stops wetting on their own. These include waterproof pants and bedding, lifting, restricting fluids, motivational techniques and medications. Because of the interplay of various factors that cause bedwetting, some children will require a combination of treatments.

Curative approaches are presently limited to bedwetting alarms. Acupuncture and chiropractic medicine are purported to have curative effects, however their role is beyond the scope of this book.

Long-term effectiveness of bedwetting solutions

Supportive	% children dry one year later
Waiting	15 %
Restricting fluids	15 %
Waking your child	15 %
Using alarm clocks	15 %
Medications*	15 %
Curative	
Bedwetting Alarms	70-80 %

*used 3-6 months

Supportive therapies

Waiting/doing nothing

A child who is younger than 6 may not be physically or emotionally mature enough to learn to stay dry at night. Waiting a few months, or even a year or two, may secure an optimal approach to bedwetting.

Waiting or doing nothing can be burdensome and stressful for everyone involved. Remember, your child cannot yet control his nighttime bedwetting. Negative remarks and punishment may hinder his progress; at the very least they won't help. Please don't be angry about the added workload; instead, try to be matter-of-fact about the burden.

Seven Steps to Nighttime Dryness

You can turn this waiting period into a learning opportunity for your child. One of the greatest burdens of bedwetting is daily laundry. He may be willing to help strip his bed linens, carry them to the washing machine and help make his bed. Here are some hints to decrease the workload:

■ Use disposable pants until your child is ready for treatment
■ Use washable, waterproof-backed pads that can be changed during the night so your child is dry as much as possible
■ Wake your child to urinate in the bathroom before you go to bed (this won't ensure dryness but it will be one less urination in the bed)
■ Use disposable waterproof pads
■ Use vinyl mattress covers that can be cleaned with disinfectant spray to decrease odor
■ Place a few pair of clean pajamas and/or underwear next to the bed to decrease middle-of-the-night clean-up time (Note: A night light in the room will reduce the need to turn on all the lights)
■ Waterproof sleeping bag liners are more easily laundered than the entire sleeping bag
■ Do not make your child sleep in a wet bed; placing a few towels over the wet area can keep your child comfortable until morning

Because some bedwetting children will spontaneously stop wetting each year, a few parents will see the problem resolve without intervention. The majority, however, will see bedwetting persist even after waiting. When you do choose to start an intervention after a period of waiting, chances are your child will be old enough to cooperate and be motivated, and/or your family will be at a more stable time in your lives. Once a child reaches 8, intervention should begin even if he doesn't seem highly motivated. Some children become motivated once they realize there is something they can do to fix the problem.

You know your child best. You'll know when the time is right to begin intervention.

Restricting fluids

Wetting often takes place not because the bladder is too full, but more likely because the pelvic floor muscles that help hold the urine in relax and allow urine to flow out. Many families have severely restricted their child's fluids after 6 p.m. and continue to see wetting two hours after their child goes to bed—even after he voided twice before bedtime. In some cases, the child sneaks drinks from the bathtub or sink because he is thirsty. Restricting fluids can become a battleground in families.

> *It's fine to let your child drink enough water*
> *after dinner to quench his thirst.*

Common sense does tell us that drinking *large* amounts in the hour or two before bed will increase the likelihood that your child will wet. Large input leads to large output! However, you should allow your child to drink some fluids—enough to quench his thirst—even up to bedtime. Allowing your child to drink water as his beverage of choice after dinner often eliminates the power struggle surrounding fluid intake. Most children do not "over-drink" water as they might other beverages. Again, some beverages such as carbonated and caffeinated drinks and citrus juices can actually increase urine production or urgency. Milk contains tryptophan, which may contribute to sleeping more soundly. (Remember grandmother's advice to drink a glass of warm milk before bedtime to help you sleep better.) These beverages should be avoided in the evening. Some medications, such as *desmopressin* (DDAVP), require a limited nighttime fluid intake to prevent fluid overload.

Waking your child at night (lifting)

Many parents ask about a technique called "lifting." Lifting means getting your child out of bed during the night and walking or carrying him to the bathroom. In some cases, this technique does provide nights of dryness. However, it is likely that your child is emptying his bladder before it's full, making it difficult to learn the proper response to the full-bladder signal. Most children have no recollection of being taken to the toilet, even though they may talk to you or look awake. Also, lifting your child at the same time each night may make his bladder used to being emptied at that time, rather than holding it until morning.

Because your child learns nothing by this method, he will wet on nights you forget to lift him. Lifting does "buy time" in some families until your child is ready for a bedwetting alarm.

If your child stays outside your home, especially with relatives or close friends, you could ask the other adults to continue this technique in your absence. If the family isn't one you could share this information with, using other protection such as disposable pants, a waterproof sleeping bag liner or medication may be necessary. Do not expect your child to be dry by himself, even if you have lifted him to the toilet each night for months or even years. He will very much depend on you to do this for him.

Using alarm clocks
Some parents have tried setting an alarm clock at a specific time each night. They wake their child but find he has already wet or may not physically need to urinate for several hours. There is no way of knowing how to predict when the proper time is. Many children do urinate when prompted to go at an arbitrary time. However, they may not remember in the morning and will not make any association between feeling the need to urinate and walking to the bathroom.

Some parents have tried setting an alarm in their child's room, but find their child doesn't respond to this sound. Most children require a louder noise to be aroused from deep sleep than adults do. Studies done by fire departments in the last few years support the common parent observation that their children sleep "very soundly."[1] The studies examined the ability of (non-bedwetting) children to respond to smoke detectors of up to 85 decibels (equivalent to a lawn mower). As much as 89 percent of children tested were not awakened by the sound. All of the adults were awakened. These same children were finally alerted by their parents' voices. We know that children's arousal from sound sleep is different from that of adults, and that arousal abilities change as children grow older. We also know that children can be conditioned to respond to familiar sounds and know how to respond to that sound.

Treating constipation

Many parents do not realize there is a close link between stool patterns and bedwetting. Constipation is defined as hard, dry and/or painful bowel movements. Parents are often aware of constipation when children are in diapers, but once the children have achieved bowel control, parents do not pay as much attention to bowel movements. Constipation or bowel problems may come to the parent's attention when there is staining in the underwear (often caused by leakage of liquid stool around a hard mass) or if there is associated abdominal pain or rectal bleeding after a particularly large stool. Painful defecation can lead to withholding stool, ignoring the body's signals to empty, more constipation and a vicious cycle.

Even more common than constipation in children is a pattern of irregular defecation. Irregular defecation is defined as bowel movements that are not daily. Because of busy schedules and school demands, children often spend eight to 10 hours per day away from home. School bathrooms are not conducive to privacy from your friends. Few children choose to have a bowel movement while at school, even if this means overriding strong urges to defecate. Once in the privacy of their home, the urge may have dissipated and your child forgets about it until the next day. If your child has enough bulk and fluids in his diet, the urges come more frequently. Your child can empty his bowel when it's convenient.

> *Your child needs the equivalent of his age plus six grams of fiber in his diet every day.*

If you closely monitor your child's stool pattern, you'll likely be genuinely surprised at his irregularity. Even if he has never complained of hard or painful stools, large stools may be passed only every three to four days. Some parents even note that their children's stools regularly plug up the plumbing!

Bedwetting and infrequent stool patterns may be linked mechanically. The bowel and bladder are closely situated in the body. An overfull bowel can decrease the bladder's ability to fully expand. The bladder contracts—even though it could still hold more urine—resulting in more frequent urination and bedwetting.

What's more, a chronically full bowel rubs against the bladder wall, gradually desensitizing your child to that "full feeling." Rubbing inhibits the transmission of impulses that tell your child's brain his bladder is full. Such decreased sensitivity can happen during the day, allowing day wetting, or during the night, increasing night wetting. Since the same nerve pathways are used for bowel and bladder, many children with wetting problems will have drastic improvement when the stool patterns are regular.

Once you've identified an irregular bowel pattern, you can help your child to defecate more regularly. A soft bowel movement every one to two days is recommended. An empty bowel allows the bladder to expand to its maximum capacity and for your child's brain to once again interpret the bladder's signals of fullness.

A high-fiber diet will help to ensure frequent soft bowel movements. Nutrition facts on packaged-food labels list fiber grams. Your child needs his age plus six grams of fiber per day.[2] Have him go through the grocery store with you and point out what he would like to include as part of his high-fiber diet. Don't forget about breakfast cereals! Cracklin' Oat Bran and Raisin Bran are two good sources of fiber that children will eat. Please note that milk and dairy products can be constipating, so substituting fruit juices and water for milk may make a difference. Finicky eaters usually tolerate fiber supplements such as Citracel Clear or Metamucil snack bars.

If your child has tried a high-fiber diet for a week or two with no noted improvement in their stool patterns, you may add a natural laxative. Please contact your health-care provider for dosage guidelines.

A regular time and place to defecate is also important. Allowing your child time and privacy is necessary for regular bowel habits. Some parents remind their children to use the bathroom after school or after dinner. Explaining the relationship between bedwetting and their infrequent stools may encourage some children to use the bathroom when the urge hits, rather than postponing it.

If daytime stool soiling in the underwear is noted, please alert your health-care provider. Treating encopresis is more involved than treating occasional constipation, so it should be directed by your pediatrician or nurse practitioner. Occasionally, children are referred to a specialist to rule out associated bowel problems. Daytime stool soiling should be addressed before tackling wetting problems.

Using medications

A few medications are indicated for children with bedwetting. Medications are designed to curb bedwetting by either decreasing the amount of urine produced at night or by allowing the bladder to hold more urine. Medication often has immediate results, but when you stop it, the relapse rate is high—about 80 percent. If you use medication for 12 weeks and stop, most children will still be wetting.

The most frequently prescribed medication for enuresis is DDAVP. This synthetic form of the natural hormone *vasopressin* decreases the quantity of urine produced for eight to 12 hours. It works quickly, usually within one hour of taking it. DDAVP allows many children to sleep dry that night, which makes it particularly useful for sleepovers and camps. DDAVP is available in two forms: a nasal spray and tablet. The tablet is preferred because it delivers a more consistent and convenient dose. Also, children with allergic congestion can get erratic results with the nasal spray. Dosage of DDAVP must be individualized, with one to three tablets (0.2 mg.) each night before bed as the recommended dose. The greatest number of dry nights is achieved by 0.4 to 0.6 mg. nightly.[3] If your child is taking the medication for a situation outside of his home, such as sleepover camp, start it ahead of time to establish the appropriate dose. Your child's doctor or nurse practitioner is responsible for determining your child's dosage, but the general recommendation is as follows:

■ If your child wets when taking one tablet, increase it to two.
■ If wetting occurs with two tablets, his dosage should be three tablets.
■ Three tablets is the maximum amount recommended for any age group.

DDAVP does not stop wetting in every child. Increasing the length of time taken will not make it work. The expected results should be seen in a week or two. Parents should realize that this medication does not provide long-lasting effects, but it does buy time.

DDAVP provides short-term dryness for many children.

DDAVP is a safe medication with very few side effects. Reported side effects include headache or water intoxication if a large amount of water is ingested after taking it.[4] The manufacturer provides fluid guidelines, recommending no more than four ounces of water before bedtime. This medication can be safely used for three- to six-month intervals with a one week break. If wetting persists, it can be used for another interval. DDAVP is expensive, as much as $4 per tablet. The cost should be taken into account when considering long-term use.

Oxybutynin (Ditropan) is another medication that can be useful in treating enuresis in some children. If your child has clinical signs of small functional bladder capacity—frequency or urgency during the day—this medication may also assist with nighttime dryness. Ditropan works by relaxing the bladder's smooth muscle, increasing bladder capacity and delaying the initial desire to void.[5] Your child's health-care provider can help you decide if this medication would be a helpful adjunct; he will determine the proper dosage. This medication is not expensive, and it's safe. Possible side effects include a dry mouth, constipation and decreased ability to sweat. Drinking daytime fluids and taking breaks to "cool off" are important in the summer.

Curative therapy
Bedwetting alarms
Bedwetting alarms help your child achieve nighttime dryness by conditioning him to stop the flow of urine when sleeping. A loud noise sounds at the first drops of urine, awakening you and your child. Over time, your child will learn to sense the need to wake up in response to a full bladder and to contract the pelvic floor muscles to inhibit the flow of urine.

We don't know exactly how bedwetting alarms work. The alarm may cause a physiological change, triggering the brain into the circadian rhythm for ADH release or teaching contraction of the pelvic floor muscles in response to a full bladder.[6] The success rate of using a bedwetting alarm approaches 80 percent, and the relapse rate is much lower than when using medication alone.

Children are 13 times more likely to achieve dryness using a bedwetting alarm than with no treatment.

A bedwetting alarm is not an alarm clock, which goes off at an arbitrary time each night to wake up your child to urinate in the toilet. Parents often comment that their child does not hear an alarm clock when it rings—either at the designated time at night or in the morning. They are very concerned that their child will not hear a bedwetting alarm. In the beginning, most children *do not* respond to the bedwetting alarm. It's more for the parents. Over time, your child develops a new response whether he remembers hearing the alarm or not.

Most alarms consist of a small, wearable plastic alarm box that attaches to the shoulder area and a moisture sensor that attaches to snug-fitting underwear. You play an important role in helping your child arouse in response to the alarm. Because of your child's decreased sleep arousal, you'll probably hear the alarm before your child responds to it. By reminding your child what to do next—walk to the bathroom to urinate—you'll help establish a new response. Over time, your child will learn to do this independently and sleep dry all night. Use of an alarm does require your time, patience and motivation, as well as your child's. Your family will experience more success if your expectations are realistic. Remember, learning a new behavior is a process that requires weeks or months, not a few days.

Permanent dryness is more likely to be achieved by having your child use the alarm until he has two consecutive weeks of dryness, then using the alarm every other night for two more weeks while maintaining dryness. Some children want to stop using the alarm after achieving a few dry nights, but stopping prematurely can lead to a relapse of wetting.

Seven Steps to Nighttime Dryness

Because bedwetting alarms offer the most effective permanent treatment for bedwetting, the rest of this book will discuss their proper use. Using enuresis alarms will benefit most children. In fact, children are 13 times more likely to achieve dryness using an alarm than with no treatment.[7] If your child doesn't improve after a few months of correct usage, you can contact your health-care provider for further recommendations.

Using medications and a bedwetting alarm together

Research indicates that the relapse rate of using an alarm and medications simultaneously is much lower than that of using medications alone. While medication can be important in the treatment of bedwetting, its effect is only temporary unless your child learns a new response to a full bladder or stops wetting spontaneously while he is taking the medication.

> *Combining medications and alarm therapy is more effective than using medications alone.*

DDAVP can be used with a bedwetting alarm, but in a lesser dosage so your child wets a smaller amount closer to morning. Many children with enuresis wet for the first time only 90 minutes to two hours after they go to bed. Since this is a particularly difficult time for independent sleep arousal to occur, moving your child's night wetting back several hours may foster success when using a bedwetting alarm. Your child's health-care provider will instruct you whether this is appropriate for your child.

Dosage is key to combining these two therapies. If the dosage of DDAVP is preventing all wetting, there would be no benefit of using an alarm because wetting is what triggers the alarm. A smaller dose of DDAVP—as little as half the dose your child needs to stay dry all night—may be enough to allow some wetting so the alarm will sound. When your child has 14 consecutive nights of dryness, the dose could be reduced again. As your child learns a new response to a full bladder— getting up or holding the urine until morning—you can gradually discontinue the medication. Because DDAVP is a short-acting medication, temporarily increasing the dosage to prevent all wetting can be useful for single-night sleepovers, camps or vacations. When your child returns home, he can resume using the alarm and taking a lower medication dosage. Combining medication and a bedwetting alarm lowers the relapse rate when the medication is discontinued.

In some situations, your child's physician may prescribe Ditropan to help maintain dryness. Even though this medication rarely prevents wetting if given by itself, it can effectively be combined with an alarm. Ditropan allows the bladder to relax, hold more urine and send less urgent messages to the brain. It allows children more time to respond to their alarms. Ditropan can also be combined with DDAVP. As your child makes progress in hearing the alarm, stopping the flow of urine and waking to go to the bathroom—ultimately having dry nights— you can gradually decrease the dosages. One tablet of Ditropan can be decreased by half by cutting on the scored line. Consult your prescribing health-care provider before adjusting your child's medication dosages (Note: The extended release preparation of *oxybutynin*, Ditropan XL, should not be cut.)

Less-common treatments

Bladder-stretching exercises. Doctors used to recommend that parents teach a bedwetting child to hold as much urine as possible during the day. The theory was "holding it" would stretch the bladder. As you can imagine, children rarely cooperated with this method because it's quite uncomfortable. What's more, children who could accomplish this during their waking hours still wet the bed! Experts now recommend that children drink enough during the day so they feel the urge to urinate every two to three hours. They should not be encouraged to hold their urine for extended periods of time. The average person urinates five to nine times a day.

Biofeedback. Biofeedback has a good track record in helping children with daytime voiding problems. The computerized information allows children to see how contracting and relaxing various pelvic and abdominal muscles relates to urination. As children achieve success in controlling daytime voiding problems, some will also achieve nighttime dryness. Biofeedback is not commonly used for primary nocturnal enuresis, however, because most of these children report no daytime voiding problems.

Alternative therapies. Alternative therapies such as acupuncture have produced some reduction in bedwetting. The number of sites needled and the frequency and length of treatments make this unappealing for many children. Chiropractors also report some success with enuresis. Children with neurological or spine problems may benefit most from chiropractic intervention. Again, frequent visits and expense make exploring this option less attractive. Hypnosis tapes also have been marketed for the treatment of bedwetting, but there is no published research on their effectiveness.

Teach your child lifelong strategies

Some adults themselves have learned strategies for staying dry by trial and error, and you can teach them to your child.

- Many parents, upon learning about the benefits of urinating twice before bedtime, report they have consistently done this for years. You can teach your child to make "double voiding" part of his lifelong bedtime routine.

- Teach your child to get out of bed and go to the bathroom when he is awakened for any reason. Some of these awakenings may be his bladder trying to send a message to a "partially asleep brain." Even an arousal to a household pet making noise or a parent getting ready for work should prompt your child to get up and use the bathroom, then go back to sleep.

- Many adults have learned not to over-drink fluids in the evening— not that they are worried about wetting, but because they prefer not to get up so frequently during the night to eliminate those fluids. Children, too, can learn to make a wise choice in amount and type of beverages they consume in the evenings. A small glass of water is a better choice than a can of soda. Especially if your child is staying outside of your home, encourage him to make wise choices.

Many adults have also learned to spread out their fluid intake over the course of a day, thus eliminating a push to quench their thirst in the evenings. Some school-aged children consume very little fluid during the day. They may have a little milk with cereal in the morning and part of a carton of milk or juice for lunch. Understandably, when they get home in the afternoon, they are very thirsty. However, if the majority of your daily fluids are consumed between 4 and 9 p.m., your body must rid itself of the wastes late in the day. Encourage your child to drink adequate fluid during the day. He can accomplish this by drinking a bottle of water or two drinks at lunchtime, along with frequent drinks from the water fountain.

References

[1] Cunningham, TM. And the Children Slept: An independent investigative study concerning reports of non-arousal by children to activated smoke detection alarms and related research. www.cfaa.cq. Dec. 2002; 1-18.

[2] Parker, PH. To Do or Not to Do? That is the Question. Pediatric Constipation. Pediatr Ann. 1999;28:283-290.

[3] Skoog SJ, Stokes A, Turner KL. Oral desmopressin: a randomized, double-blind placebo-controlled trial of effectiveness in children with primary nocturnal enuresis. J Urol. 1997;158:1035-1040.

[4] DDAVP Tablets, product information. Bridgewater, NJ, Aventis Pharmaceuticals Products Inc, 2001.

[5] Ditropan, product information. Mountain View, CA, ALZA Corporation, 1998.

[6] Harari M, Moulden A. Personal Practice. Nocturnal Enuresis: What is happening? J Paediatr Child Health. 2000; 36:78-81.

[7] Bosson S, Lyth N. Nocturnal enuresis. In Barton S, ed. Clinical Evidence. Issue 5. London: BMJ Publishing; 2001; 6:300-305.

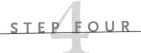

Choose a
bedwetting alarm

A bedwetting (enuresis) alarm is a device designed to teach your child to respond to a full bladder by using the toilet during the night. It's essentially a middleman—something to alert your child that she is in the process of wetting until her brain and her bladder learn to talk to each other at night.

Unlike an alarm clock that is set to arbitrarily awaken your child to urinate in the toilet or you getting her up at scheduled times, the bedwetting alarm responds to your child's biological need to urinate—the timing and amount of which will vary from night to night. Bedwetting alarms are based on classic behavior modification theory, which was first noted with Pavlov's dogs. Bedwetting alarms are a mainstay in enuresis treatment, and they are an easy first step for parents to employ.

Jill's Story

Jill is 12 and has tried several methods of overcoming her bedwetting. Her parents bought her a vibrating-only enuresis alarm. When she failed to awake to it, they decided that alarms would not work for her. Another time they set her alarm clock for every two hours. Sometimes, she was already wet when it went off. A prescription medication that her doctor recommended did not keep her dry that night. What can Jill do?

Alarms come in several different types and styles. The most common alarm is a wearable alarm.

A *wearable alarm* consists of a sensor, an alarm unit and often, a cord that connects the two. The sensor is usually attached to the area of her underwear or pajamas that will receive the first drop of urine; it senses moisture and makes a noise loud enough to wake up you and her. With your help at first, she'll get up and use the toilet. After a few months of

Wearable alarm

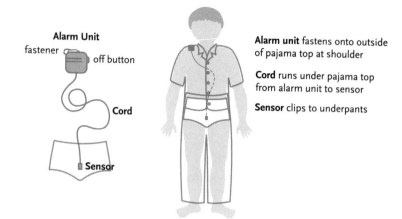

Alarm Unit
fastener
off button
Cord
Sensor

Alarm unit fastens onto outside of pajama top at shoulder

Cord runs under pajama top from alarm unit to sensor

Sensor clips to underpants

Bell-and-pad alarm

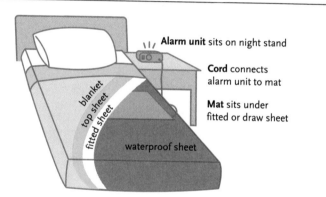

Alarm unit sits on night stand

Cord connects alarm unit to mat

Mat sits under fitted or draw sheet

blanket
top sheet
fitted sheet
waterproof sheet

Wireless alarm

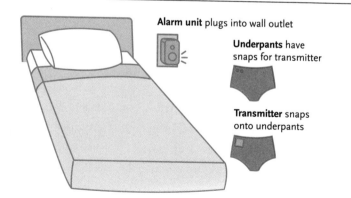

Alarm unit plugs into wall outlet

Underpants have snaps for transmitter

Transmitter snaps onto underpants

associating the alarm with the need to go to the bathroom, your child's brain will begin to understand the feeling of a full bladder and, ultimately, wake her up to urinate before the alarm goes off.

Bell-and-pad alarms work like they sound: Your child sleeps on a firm plastic pad. When she wets, the urine leaks onto the pad and an alarm sounds. This type of alarm requires a larger amount of urine to trigger the alarm. If your child rolls off the pad or doesn't wet a large amount, the alarm won't sound. What's more, some children find the size and texture of this alarm uncomfortable.

Wireless alarms consist of special underwear with sensor strips sewn in place, a small transmitter snapped on the waist and a remote alarm. Moisture triggers the transmitter to sound an alarm that's plugged into the wall. The child or parent must walk to the wall alarm to turn it off, therefore getting someone out of bed. Drawbacks to this type of alarm: the special underwear must fit properly and be ready each night.

Alarm basics

A common myth is bedwetting alarms are useless for deep-sleeping children. Remember that almost all children with bedwetting sleep more soundly than their peers who don't wet. (However, not all sound-sleeping children have bedwetting.) Initially, you play an important part in arousing your sleeping child once the alarm has gone off. When most children hear the alarm tested when they are awake, they can't believe they could possibly sleep through that loud sound. But most bedwetting children do not initially wake up to the loud—80 decibel—alarm at first. For this reason, you usually will hear the alarm first, even if your child's room is down the hall. (If you and your child sleep on different floors, it's wise to use a baby monitor during this time.)

Once you hear the alarm, you should respond quickly to your child. If she is sitting up or moving in response to the noise, just remind her what to do next—go to the bathroom. If she is still sleeping soundly, you may gently shake her, call her name, turn on the light or do whatever else it takes to arouse her and take her to the bathroom.

It is absolutely necessary to use an audible alarm with all children at first because you need the loud sound to alert you to the first drops of wetness so you can help your child. A vibratory alarm doesn't let you help your child respond to the alarm because you won't feel it vibrate. In fact, parents who have tried a vibratory alarm report their children sleep through it and wake up wet with no idea of what they could have done differently.

To get the best response, use an audible alarm so you can help your child.

To be effective, the alarm must work every time. That means you or your child must attach it in the correct place on her clothing, and it must remain attached all night. Alarms may falter for some common reasons.

■ Some children will unintentionally pull off the alarm or otherwise disconnect it as their first response to the sound—and often before you hear it. Your child then wakes up wet with a disconnected alarm.

■ Alarms with metal snaps can come off if your child sleeps restlessly or if you attach it to clothing that is too thick.

■ If the alarm isn't placed where it can sense the first drop of urine, the clothing would have to be saturated before the alarm responds.

When you select an alarm, make sure it attaches firmly to your child's clothing. Have your child dressed in snug-fitting panties or briefs, not loose pajamas or boxer shorts. And be as precise as possible when determining where to attach the alarm, then actually attaching it.

Key criteria for choosing an alarm

If you have decided to use a bedwetting alarm to help your child achieve dryness, the key to success is choosing the right one. Although most alarms sense moisture and respond by making a sound and/or vibration, there are many differences in the various models.

Before purchasing an alarm, consider the following criteria:

Usability

- Will your child wear an alarm in the first place?
- Is the alarm too big or too small for your child's size?
- Are you willing and able to sew sensor pockets onto underwear, or do you need a clip-on sensor that fastens to any pair of underwear?
- Will you be sure the designated underwear is laundered and ready to go at bedtime?
- Which alarm would you be most likely to use if you were your child? Look for a "kid cool" design to encourage your child to use it.

Comfort

- Is the alarm lightweight and comfortable to wear? Children generally won't wear alarms with bulky moisture pads. Younger children, especially, are more comfortable using little alarms with little sensors— some are smaller than a postage stamp so kids barely feel them if they're placed correctly.

Durability

- Are the sensors and alarm made of durable material with few metal parts to rust?
- Is the alarm unit watertight to prevent urine seepage if it is placed in the underwear?
- Are replacement parts readily available so that you can use the alarm for more than one child, if necessary?
- Are cleaning directions included?
- Does the alarm carry a manufacturer's warranty?

Connection

- Is the sensor difficult to unhook during sleep movements? Be leery of alarms that use metal snaps and hooks that easily come undone.
- If the sensor does become unhooked, does it alert the wearer?

Sound

- Does the alarm sound to wake your sleeping child? While combination sound/vibration alarms add an extra dimension of arousal, alarms that only vibrate won't wake the majority of bedwetting children. Initially it is important that you can hear the alarm to help your child get up. Most alarms sound at 80 to 90 decibels when placed in the manufacturer's recommended site. Some bedside units make louder sounds because they are not in such close proximity to your child's ear.
- Where is the sound unit located? It should be close to your child's ear or close on the bedside. Make sure it isn't muffled by blankets.
- How is the sound unit attached?
- Does your child need to wear a T-shirt, and is this acceptable to her?

Turnoff

- Once the alarm sounds, how is it turned off?
- Can your child easily disconnect the sensor and go back to sleep? An alarm that takes more than one step to turn off promotes more alertness, and it gives you enough time to hear the alarm and get to your child's room.

Special needs

- Does your child have special needs that make one type of alarm more appealing?
- Is the feeling of a sensor attached to her underwear something she objects to? Maybe a pad-type alarm, where nothing is actually attached to her body or clothing, is best.
- Has she tried a certain type of alarm in the past and needs a change? Some children with special needs find the alarm sound or tone objectionable. Your child may prefer a recordable alarm, where a favorite voice or sound is used. Some families choose to use an alarm to alert them when their special needs child should be changed.

The following table applies these criteria to the common alarms found on the market:

Comparison of various alarms

Brand	Rating	Sound	Sensor	Usability	Turnoff	Warranty	Cost	Comments
Wearable alarms								
Malem Ultimate	6	●	●	●	●	● 1 year	●	Multiple colors/tones, 2-step turnoff, sound and vibration
Malem	6	●	●	●	●	● 1 year	●	Multiple colors/tones, 2-step turnoff
Wet-Stop	4	●	●	○	○	● 1 year	●	Cloth pouches sewn on underwear
SleepDry	3	●	○	○	○	● 1 year	●	
DRI Sleeper	2	●	○	○	○	○ 60 days	●	Sensor worn in panty liner
Nite Train-r	2	●	○	○	○	○ 60 days	●	Large pads worn inside underwear
Nytone	2	●	○	○	○	○ 30 days	●	Heavy, worn on wrist
Potty Pager	1	○	○	○	○	○ 90 days	●	No sound, vibration only
Pad-type alarms								
Wet Call	3	●	○	○	●	○ 60 days	●	
Malem	3	●	○	○	●	● 1 year	○	Variable volume
Wireless alarms								
Rodger BAS	5	●	●	●	●	● 1 year	○	

● Meets criteria
○ Does not meet criteria

Rating Criteria:
Sound—Does the unit emit a loud tone to alert both parent and child?
Sensor—Does the unit have a comfortable, easy to use attachment that quickly detects moisture and stays securely attached?
Usability—Is the unit lightweight, easy to set up and reattach during the night? Can children easily use the alarm?
Turnoff—Does the unit prevent children from simply tugging on or removing the sensor to quickly stop the alarm?
Warranty—Children, on average, require 12 weeks to attain dryness. Is the warranty period for more than 90 days?
Cost—Does the unit cost less than $100?

Source: Manufacturer Information 2003. • See www.bedwettinghandbook.com for updated product and purchase information.

Where to purchase an alarm

Because bedwetting alarms are specialized items, general pharmacies or stores with children's supplies rarely stock them. Specialized catalogs and online stores carry the most extensive supply. The Bedwetting Store (www.bedwettingstore.com) offers a comprehensive selection of bedwetting alarms, as well as other items that families with bedwetting children might need. Alarms from most major manufacturers can be purchased here, including Malem, Malem Ultimate, Wet-Stop, DRI Sleeper, Nite Train-r, Nytone, Wet Call and others. It is worthwhile to visit this web site or look through the store's catalog to choose an alarm that best suits your child's needs. Products like waterproof bedding, waterproof sleeping bag liners and urine removal cleaners can be found here.

The Bedwetting Store 1-800-214-9605
www.bedwettingstore.com

Some alarm manufacturers also sell their own products. You can contact them directly if you require specific products.

Alarms range in price from $60 to $200, depending on features and design. They can typically be purchased for less than $100. Many families find that the money they save on disposable pants and laundry quickly pays for the alarm.

A few insurance companies consider bedwetting alarms to be pieces of durable medical equipment (DME). Check with your insurance carrier to see if an alarm is a covered benefit.

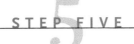

Prepare to use your bedwetting alarm

Consistent, effective use of your bedwetting alarm is the key to your child achieving nighttime dryness. While alarms offer a long-term, permanent cure for bedwetting, they do not offer an instantaneous cure. It will take a little time and conditioning for your child to respond to the alarm at all, and longer for him to stay completely dry. Before you even begin to use the alarm, you'll need to prepare yourself, your child and his environment for the endeavor of becoming consistently dry.

Adam's Story

Adam and his parents are all set. They picked out his new bedwetting alarm and everyone is excited to begin. The first night, Adam did not hear the alarm and had already wet by the time his dad got to his room. Should this have happened?

Prepare yourself

It's up to you to set realistic expectations for yourself, your child and anyone else affected by this process. It takes 10 to 12 weeks for the average child to be consistently dry; some may take longer. What's more, it is rare for a child to hear the alarm and walk to the bathroom alone the first night. Such behavior is a learned response, and learning requires parent participation. Don't be disappointed in your child or yourself when accidents happen over the course of his learning to stay dry.

The first month will be difficult. Some success is possible in the first week, if your child is excited and doesn't sleep as soundly as usual. In some cases, the second week is more difficult as you and your child relax and more wetting takes place. If you ensure your child is not overly tired when he goes to bed, you'll help his progress.

Get to know your alarm

Now that you have decided to treat your child's bedwetting with an
alarm, read the manufacturer's instructions for use and maintenance.
Make sure you have an extra set of batteries; low batteries are the most
common reason why alarms stop working.

Allow your child to visually inspect and play with the alarm— turn it
off and on a few times—to help him be comfortable with the sound it
makes. Some manufacturers, such as Malem, use sounds that remind
kids of electronic games. Most alarms have a decibel level of 80 to 90,
a safe level given the alarm's close proximity to your child's ear. Adults
typically arouse to sounds of 40 to 50 decibels.

If you've selected a pad-type alarm, you'll need a moist cloth to test it.
Place the cloth on the pad so it's touching two strips simultaneously.
Apply adequate pressure and the alarm will sound; some alarms are
sensitive only to moisture and pressure at the same time.

Prepare your child

Your child may be a bit apprehensive about using the alarm, even if he's
excited about the prospect of staying dry all night. Reassure him that the
alarm won't hurt him in any way; it is only a noise or vibration to
remind him in the night to get out of bed and urinate. Many children
(and adults) think the alarm is loud and may be frightening during the
night. That is rarely the case. Since most children with bedwetting have
a decreased arousal from sleep, many don't hear the alarm at all at first.
Even if they do, the sound shouldn't scare them if they know what it is.
Allow siblings and other household members to hear the alarm. Tell
them they may hear the sound during the night. If they do, they do not
need to respond and should go back to sleep. Even siblings who share a
room are rarely bothered by the alarm.

Be sure to take a trial run while your child is still awake on the first
night. He should dress in his nightwear, hook up the alarm and cause
the alarm to sound. Encourage him to practice each step of his response
to the alarm's sound. For example, "I'll get out of bed, turn off my alarm
and walk to the bathroom. Then I'll change into clean underwear, reat-

tach my alarm and go back to bed." Your child will need your help in the beginning, but it's important that he can verbalize and act out the expected behavior.

Have your child practice what he will do when the alarm sounds.

Prepare your child's room

To help your child get out of bed and to the bathroom in the dark of night, you must prepare his room. A nightlight in the bathroom will help direct him to the proper place to empty his bladder. It's not uncommon that children with bedwetting will also have "sleepwalking," and they'll urinate in the closet or a hamper, mistakenly thinking that they are in the bathroom. For this reason, it is important for you to be sure your child actually gets to the bathroom when the alarm sounds. Another small nightlight in your child's room can give you enough light to change bedding and underwear without turning on all the lights.

If your child routinely sleeps in a top bunk bed, make other temporary sleeping arrangements. Have him switch beds with his sibling, or lay his mattress on the floor so he can more easily walk to the bathroom during the night.

Parents must be able to hear the alarm from their room.

To give your child the help he'll need, you must be able to hear your child's bedwetting alarm when it sounds. Typically, unless you are an extremely sound sleeper, you can hear the alarm from a room down the hall. If you and your child sleep on separate floors or down a long hall from each other, it's wise to use a baby monitor. You may feel you need to sleep in your child's room until you see what his response is, but if you can respond quickly when the alarm sounds, this won't be necessary. If you and your partner are very sound sleepers and absolutely cannot respond to the alarm from your room, you may wish to temporarily move to your child's room; this would be better than having your child move to your room so he can get used to his nighttime traffic pattern.

Prepare your child's nightclothes

Now is the time to stop using disposable pants or diapers at night and move your child to cloth underwear. Most alarms work more effectively when attached to cloth than to plastic or the ultra-absorbent materials in diapers. What's more, your child can more readily track his progress if he's in underwear; he can watch his urine spots shrink from the size of two basketballs to the size of a baseball, and eventually to a drop on his underwear. Being able to watch this change will help him develop his new behavior of holding his urine and emptying it in the toilet.

Clothes for wearable alarms

Choosing proper underwear is important. Close-fitting briefs work best for both boys and girls. Boxers and baggy pajama bottoms allow too much space between the urine being excreted and the sensor. And if the urine flow is directed away from the moisture sensor, the alarm won't sound until a large spot of wetness occurs. Close-fitting briefs help eliminate these obstacles.

Attach the alarm to close-fitting cloth underwear.

If your alarm requires pouches to be sewn to the underwear for correct sensor placement, have your child try on the underwear first. Position the pouch so the sensor will most likely sense the first drop of moisture. For young girls, this would be in the crotch area of the panties. If your daughter sleeps regularly on her back, the pouch might be positioned a little further back than if she sleeps mostly on her side or belly. If your alarm doesn't require pouch placement, your child can easily adjust the sensor's position on his underwear. Remind him to place it in an area that is most likely to get wet with the first drop of urine. Do not place the sensor at or around the waistband or leg openings, which are uncomfortable positions that won't sense moisture quickly. You can experiment with different sensor placements until you find the optimal position.

Most alarm units attach to the shoulder of a pajama top or T-shirt. Some children who prefer to sleep with no shirt may temporarily need to wear a lightweight shirt. You may attach the alarm unit to any top, even a sleeveless undershirt. Shoulder placement puts the sound close to your child's ear so he can hear it easier and keeps bedding and blankets from interfering with the alarm. It's a comfortable placement that allows your child to turn over without feeling the alarm. Be sure to follow your alarm manufacturer's instructions for where to place the alarm unit.

Some alarms units and sensors are attached to each other with a thin plastic cord. Be sure to place the cord under your child's shirt so the alarm moves with him, decreasing the opportunity for his body movement to pull on the alarm.

Clothes for pad-type alarms

A pad-type alarm consists of a moisture-sensing pad, which your child lays on, and an alarm unit, which you usually place on a bedside table or near the head of the bed. When your child urinates, the pad senses the moisture and triggers the alarm.

Your child may choose to wear a nightgown or T-shirt, with or without underwear. Obviously, disposable pants can't be used with this type of alarm. To secure the pad in place and prevent false sounding due to perspiration, place a draw-sheet (a bed sheet folded lengthwise) over it.

Prepare your child's bed

Most children who wet the bed are accustomed to wearing waterproof disposable pants at night to keep their beds dry. When you begin alarm therapy, you'll have many nights when your child wets a large amount of fluid in the bed. Everyone begins this way—there is no avoiding this step! However, you can lighten your laundry load and protect your mattress and bedding from excessive urine. Several products are available to this end.

- A fitted, vinyl waterproof mattress cover usually encases the mattress and zips in place. These covers also protect your child from allergens. In the morning, you clean the cover with a spray disinfectant and dry it off.

- A waterproof mattress pad provides absorbency as well as moisture protection. Some mattress pads will hold up to six cups of fluid. Typically, these are fitted to the mattress size and are machine washable. Because of the waterproof feature, they take longer to dry than a regular mattress pad.

- Waterproof mattress overlays are quilted, soft pieces of fabric with a waterproof layer that protect the sheets from moisture. They come in different sizes to fit your child's bed. The saddle style mattress overlay, best-suited for twin or full mattresses, has side flaps that tuck between your child's mattress and box spring to hold the pad in place. Mattress overlays can be machine washed and dried and can decrease the overall laundry load significantly.
- Disposable pads are also convenient. However, they are lightweight and are easily dislodged by your child's movement during sleep. You can secure them to your child's bed with thick tape. Some disposable pads also have adhesive strips.

Regardless of the type of protection you use, it's important that your child sleeps on a clean, dry surface. Start each night with a clean bed. Once he has urinated, be sure to replace wet items with dry ones. Remember to check and replace his top sheet or blanket if either becomes wet. As your child progresses with the alarm, the wet spots become smaller and soiling the top covers becomes less of a problem.

Create a record-keeping system

Record keeping is an important part of achieving nighttime dryness. I believe record keeping is so crucial that I have included charts and directions for recording your child's progress at the end of this book. You'll track the times your child's alarm goes off, the sizes of wet spots on the bed, deviations in food and fluid intake.

It's important to take time each morning to jot down the previous night's occurrences. If you don't, you will be faced with the difficult task of reconstructing what actually happened over several nights or weeks. Often, it's difficult enough to remember what happened just *last* night!

Tracking the times your child's alarm goes off and the sizes of the wet spots is critical for detecting patterns of wetness as well as assessing progress. Your child may begin with having large wet spots several times each night, or with alarms sounding early in the sleep cycle. Over time, you may note that his wetting episodes diminish, or his alarm goes off at a different time. You may note increased wetting on nights of athletic events, or nights when he's ill. Patterns, such as wetting toward the weekend as fatigue increases, may become evident.

You've already learned that the foods and fluids your child ingests may make a difference in the time and amount of wetting. By observing and tracking deviations in normal patterns and recording what food or fluid was different on a given night, you may be able to pinpoint food sensitivities. For example, one teenage girl noted that ice cream before bed increased her wetting episodes. By changing to sherbet or having ice cream earlier in the day, she was able to curtail her wet nights. This information was especially helpful when she planned to spend the night with friends.

Having a visual record of your child's progress can also be a potential motivator for him. Because he'll have a gradual response to his alarm, he may get impatient or tired of wearing it. Going over your records with him may encourage him to continue. For example, pointing out how large or frequent the spots were in the beginning will reassure your child that he is making progress, even if it seems slow.

Create a reward system

Because record keeping is so motivational, further refining this with the use of meaningful stars or stickers is beneficial. Younger children, ages 6 to 9 especially, respond to visual rewards such as stickers.

Cooperation and dry night stickers are helpful in younger children.

Create a weekly progress chart, kept in a place where your child will see it often, to visually display stickers received for cooperating and for having dry nights. (You can find an example of this chart on the next page, and weekly progress charts in Appendix C that you can fill out.) Each morning, your child should award himself a sticker, based on what occurred the previous night. Two categories of stars or stickers are helpful:

Cooperation stickers—perhaps colored stars or, less desirable stickers of another type. Your child earns these even if he doesn't have a dry night. In order to earn a cooperation star, he must do three things:

1. **Double void before bed.** Double voiding means urinating 20 to 30 minutes before bedtime and again immediately before lights out. Because the bladder fills at the rate of about 1 ml per minute, about an ounce of urine will be produced in 30 minutes. If your child empties this small amount of urine in the toilet, it is one ounce less to be emptied in his bed.
2. **Hook up his alarm without complaining.** You may help him, if necessary.
3. **Cooperate with you in the middle of the night.** Your child should comply when you remind him to get out of bed and go to the bathroom, change into dry underwear and re-attach the alarm.

Dry night stickers—perhaps can be gold or silver stars or a favorite type of sticker. These are earned for dry nights, accomplished when he anticipates the alarm and gets up to urinate, or when he sleeps dry all night.

As weeks go by, your child will initially see many cooperation stickers with a sprinkling of dry night stickers. Over time, you'll note more dry night stickers on consecutive nights. Making a game out of how many consecutive dry nights he has or how many dry night stickers he earns in a two- to four-week period of time is fun. Comparing the second month's chart with first month's is usually encouraging as well.

For older kids, having dry nights seems to be reward enough. However, it is still important to praise and provide incentives for their cooperation, perhaps with special time spent with you. Remember, your child cannot initially control whether he'll have a dry night so rewarding him only for dry nights can be frustrating for him. Cooperation is the key in the beginning.

This sample demonstrates how to fill out your progress chart. A blank chart that can be reproduced is in Appendix C.

Weekly progress chart

Date	Wore Alarm	Double Voided	Nighttime Cooperation	Dry Night	Woke Before Alarm	Woke to Alarm	Time of Alarm	Size of Spot S–M–L	Notes/Contributing Factors
MON 5/12	✓	✓	✓ = ★			✓	2:45	M	
TUE 5/13	✓	✓	✓ = ★	★	✓				
WED 5/14	✓	✓	✓ = ★			✓	12:30 5:45	L S	Late night soda after dinner
THU 5/15									
FRI 5/16									
SAT 5/17									
SUN 5/18									

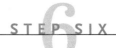

STEP SIX

Use the alarm until your child is consistently dry

By now, you know how your alarm works, and everyone is ready to begin using it. You have protected your child's bed, and you have extra underwear, pajamas, sheets and sheet protection at your child's bedside. Nightlights are installed, and you know you can hear the alarm from your bedroom. Your child, with or without your help, has attached the alarm properly. You're ready to go!

Double void before bedtime

Your child should urinate in the toilet when you tell him it's time for bed, then complete his usual nighttime ritual: brush his teeth, put on pajamas, read a story, get his clothes ready for the next day, etc. Before the lights go out, he should try to urinate once more *even if he doesn't feel like he needs to.* Remember, double voiding is one of the three requirements for "cooperation rewards" in the morning.

Respond to the alarm

Jenny's story

Jenny connects her alarm before going to bed, and she is very excited about the prospect of learning to stay dry. She double voids and goes to bed at 9 p.m. as usual. At 10:30, her parents are surprised to hear her alarm sounding; they haven't even been to bed yet. Jenny has been asleep for only an hour and a half—how can she be wetting already? After she empties her bladder in the toilet, her alarm does not sound the rest of the night. In the morning, Jenny doesn't remember being awakened by the alarm and is excited because she thinks she had a dry night.

It's likely that, at first, your child's alarm will sound within 90 minutes to two hours after her bedtime. It's not that her bladder is so full it can't hold any more, but rather that she hasn't learned to contract her

Seven Steps to Nighttime Dryness

pelvic floor muscles during sound sleep to stop her urine flow. As she learns this new response, incidents of urination within an hour or two of bedtime rapidly decrease. And as she is able to hold her urine until closer to the morning hours, she'll more easily alert to the alarm and remember it in the morning.

Regardless of when you hear your child's bedwetting alarm sound, it is critical that you respond promptly. Go to your child's room and note her response to the alarm. Don't turn off the alarm until her feet are on the floor. If necessary, wake her up by saying her name, gently shaking her or using other methods that traditionally awaken her. Remind her of the next step: "Put your feet on the floor and walk to the bathroom." You may need to help her put her legs over the side of her bed and stand up. Depending on your child's age and degree of wakefulness, you may also need to accompany her to the bathroom. When she's finished emptying her bladder, she must get into dry clothes and bedding. Help her as necessary.

Don't be discouraged if your child has no recollection of the alarm and subsequent bathroom visit in the morning— especially those trips that happen right after she falls asleep. Even if she doesn't remember, learning is still taking place.

Justin's story

Justin goes to bed at his usual time, after attaching his alarm and double voiding. He awakens to a vague, loud noise, but doesn't know what it is until his parents remind him. His parents comment that he was covering his ears and trying to pull the blankets over his head when they got to his room.

By day your child may voice understanding of his alarm, the noise it makes and what his action should be. It is very different for him, however, to hear the alarm during the night and know immediately what to do. This is why what you do is so important. By reminding your child in a calm, matter of fact manner what he should do, you facilitate a new conditioned response—one your child can accomplish without much cognitive thought. "That's your alarm. You need to go to the bathroom.

Put your feet on the floor. Let's go," is appropriate to tell him. Your child will not initially be able to think through his actions by himself. Over time, he'll respond quicker.

> Initially, your child will have emptied his bladder by the time he hears the alarm (or you respond). Over time, your child will learn to stop the urine flow when the alarm sounds. Many alarms sound when they sense even a tiny amount of urine. Eventually, your child will have only a small spot of urine on his underwear.

John's story

John connects his alarm at bedtime and goes to sleep at 10 p.m. His alarm sounds at midnight. At that time, he has a large spot of urine on his bed, but he still walks into the bathroom to attempt to urinate in the toilet. Only a few drops come out. His parents help him change into dry underwear, reconnect the alarm and change the bedding. His alarm sounds again at 5 a.m. At this time, his parents notice a medium sized spot on the bed and he has urine left to empty in the toilet. He has no recollection of the first waking, but remembers the second waking.

Initially, your child may urinate more than once each night. For this reason, it is important to connect the alarm at bedtime and after each wetting episode. This way, you can track and record each episode of urination. Your child may wet a second time only a few minutes before he wakes up in the morning. He may report he dreamed he was in the bathroom urinating in the toilet. Having the alarm sound reminds your child in this sleep state to stop the flow and get out of bed. As your child makes progress, the number of nightly episodes will decrease, and the first episode of wetting will occur closer to morning when it is easier to alert your child.

"The honeymoon period"

Katie's story

Katie attaches her alarm at bedtime and is a little nervous and excited about using it for the first time. She notices it takes a little longer than usual to go to sleep. She wakes up several times during the night to check the alarm placement and whether it has gone off yet. She stays dry all night the first few nights. On the fifth night, Katie attains her usual level of sleep, and her alarm sounds, reminding her that she needs to get up and go to the bathroom. She is disappointed that she had a wet night.

In a few cases, children have a few dry nights the very first week of using the bedwetting alarm. We call this "the honeymoon period." Because using the alarm is new and exciting, your child may not sleep as soundly as usual, and you may be very vigilant about hearing the alarm and getting to her room immediately. Typically, this phase is short-lived. By the second week, the alarm is not as exciting and children resume their normal sleep patterns. You may be concerned that the increased number of wet nights during the second week are signs of "relapse," but they are actually a more normal predictor of your child's response to the alarm. Consider these to be nights of learning. Remind your child that it is beneficial for the alarm to sound during the learning phase and not to be discouraged if she wets more during the second week than the first week. The pattern of gradually increasing dry nights will begin to evolve over the next weeks.

Signs of progress

Many families want to know if they are "on the right track"—whether their child is making the right kind of progress. Because each child will proceed at his own rate, it's difficult to say how long it will take to achieve dryness. Occasionally, a child will hear the alarm the first night and know what to do. A child with this pattern usually responds quickly, first by his independent response, then by stopping the flow of urine within the first few drops, then by anticipating the alarm or holding his urine until morning. Children in this category are rare but often progress to dryness in two to four weeks. Some children with intermittent wetting (wetting a few times per week rather than nightly) may fall into this category.

More typically, children respond to the alarm with a gradual increase of dry nights over a few weeks. Initially, your child may continue to wet nightly and have little, if any, independent response to the alarm. Do not be discouraged! Occasionally, children achieve dryness but never remember being awakened or responding to the alarm. You both can observe small steps along the path to dryness. It is important to track your child's response along the way.

> *Track your child's progress by frequency of wetting episodes, size of the wet spot, time of wetting and number of dry nights.*

Decrease in frequency of wetting episodes

During the first month, most children see a decrease in the frequency of wetting episodes. Some children never wet more than once per night, but others will, especially younger kids who regularly used disposable pants. Multiple wetting episodes are initially exhausting for parents, who have more difficulty getting back to sleep than their child does. It may help to alternate nights "on duty" with your partner or to split up the night duties—one person takes care of your child while the other strips and remakes the bed. Some parents also share the duty by dividing the night in half: one parent responds to the first wetting and the other responds to the second. Again, reminding yourself that multiple wetting episodes are temporary may help with fatigue.

Keeping good records will allow you and your child to observe this decrease in wetting episodes. For example, on nights one through 10, the alarm went off at 11:30 p.m. and 4 a.m. On nights 11 and 12, the alarm only went off at 2 a.m. For a few more nights, double wetting episodes occurred, followed by several nights of a single, later episode. This is called progress. Be sure to congratulate your child!

Smaller urine spot on the bed

Wearable bedwetting alarms sound at the first few drops of moisture. Initially, your child's alarm will sound, and you'll find he has completely emptied his bladder. Remember, this is the only response he's familiar with. The urine spot on his bed or protective pad will be large, often as big as two basketballs. Over a few weeks' time, your child will learn to stop the flow of urine when the alarm sounds, and you'll notice smaller and smaller urine spots. Once he achieves this behavior, your laundry burden will decrease significantly because only his underwear will be damp. Congratulate your child when he learns to stop his flow in response to the alarm.

A note about pad-type alarms: Your child may take longer to respond to this type of alarm. That's because his position on the pad when he urinates influences when the alarm will sound. If he's on his stomach, he'll urinate directly on the sensor, so it should sound to a few drops of urine. However, if he's on his back, a larger amount of urine must leak down to the sensor pad before it will sound. Because it's harder to stop the flow of urine once his bladder has been partially emptied (as opposed to after a drop or two has been released), it may take your child longer to learn to contract his pelvic floor muscles to stop urinating in response to the alarm. Your child may respond faster if he doesn't wear underwear to bed.

A shift in the time your child wets

As previously mentioned, many children begin by having a large wetting episode a couple of hours after bedtime. Gradually, you will notice that your child's first wetting episode occurs later in the night as he progresses with the bedwetting alarm. The later the wetting episode occurs, the more easily aroused your child will be. He may even remember hearing the alarm and walking to the bathroom. Having only one wetting episode closer to morning is certainly a sign of progress.

More consecutive dry nights

Initially, your child may have an occasional night where he is completely dry, preceded and followed by a string of wet nights. You may ask yourself what your child did differently to achieve that dry night, and you may never determine the cause. Soon, your child will have more frequent dry nights. This natural progression is rarely one of "all or nothing." Most children will have dry nights interspersed with wet nights for a few weeks. But when reviewing your records, you will note more dry nights in a row and more dry nights each week.

Some children do experience a pattern of dryness when they have a regular nightly routine, a normal dinner hour and are in good health. Illness, fatigue, a change in schedule (like vacations or summer) and evening sports activities may cause an increase in wetting. In most cases, this increase just indicates that you should use the alarm a little longer until these events do not affect your child's wetting episodes. Some families can predict the nights most likely to be wet and make sure the alarm is in place at bedtime. Intermittent use of medication, such as DDAVP, may be helpful when your child is at high risk of embarrassment if he wets, and you have not yet confirmed his reliability in staying dry.

Scott's story

Scott is a teenager who usually goes to bed around 10:30 p.m. and gets up by 6 a.m. for school. On school days, his bedwetting alarm may sound at 5:45 am, just minutes before his regular alarm clock sounds. He can usually stop his flow of urine and empty the remaining urine in the toilet. He easily recalls these episodes. On weekends, he catches up on missed rest by sleeping late, often until noon. He has noticed that his bedwetting alarm still goes off around 6 a.m. on those days. He gets up to urinate, and then goes back to bed for a few more hours of sleep.

Because of normal body rhythms, sleeping late on a weekend doesn't stop your body from urinating on a regular schedule. Remind your child of this! Also, getting up to urinate doesn't mean that you have to stay awake. Your child can easily go back to sleep. Instruct your child to make a trip to the bathroom regardless of the reason they wake up during the night. Waking to respond to a pet or a sibling, or even to visit your bedroom, can actually be your child's bladder signaling it needs to be emptied. Once he empties his bladder, he'll sleep restfully.

> *70 to 80 percent of children achieve dryness using a bedwetting alarm alone, but time and consistency improve outcome.*

When you use a bedwetting alarm, you must be patient and persevere. Seventy to 80 percent of children can achieve permanent dryness with this method, but like any type of behavioral conditioning, time and consistency improve outcome. Judging your own child's progress by looking at statistics or anecdotal stories can be counterproductive. If he is progressing in the above categories—slowly but surely—he is "on the right track."

Troubleshooting

If your child is not beginning to respond to the alarm by having smaller spots of wetness or decreasing the frequency of wetting episodes, here are several items to check.

- Make sure the alarm is working properly: it is reliably sounding each time your child wets. If it isn't, make sure the batteries are good and the battery compartment is dry. Weak batteries—the most common cause of alarm malfunction—can reduce sensor sensitivity. Be sure to clean the sensor regularly with soap and water because urine residue can cause erratic behavior. Make sure the sensor cord is smooth, intact and has no evidence of breakage.

- Make sure the sensor is positioned in the best place for detecting moisture. Remember that close fitting underwear, not boxers, pajama bottoms or disposable pants, are recommended so the sensors detect the first few drops of urine.

- Be sure you're using the alarm every night. If you use it for a few nights, then don't for a few nights, it will take your child longer to become dry. You will likely see more wetting on nights when you don't have the energy to help your child hook up his alarm. If your child goes between households, adults in both places should know how to use the alarm; have your child pack it in his overnight bag. If a special situation arises, such as vacation or camp, your child could temporarily use medication or disposable pants with the understanding he will return to using the alarm every night when he returns home.

- Make sure your child is not somehow disconnecting the alarm before you have a chance to respond and remind him about his proper response. Some children are very adept at quickly disconnecting the alarm, rolling over, going back to sleep and not recalling their actions. In this case, you might use duct tape or an extra safety pin in a strategic location to make the alarm more difficult to disconnect. Or, have your child wear an extra pair of underwear with the alarm sensor sandwiched between the two.

- If your child is using a pad type alarm, make sure he is able to stay on the pad all night. If he sleeps in a full-size bed, adjusting his sleep space so he can sleep only on the part of the bed with the alarm pad is helpful. If the alarm pad seems sensitive to body moisture, placing a towel, then a draw sheet (a sheet folded lengthwise, and placed over the pad with the edges tucked between the mattress and box spring) may help. Also, static electricity from fluffy, acrylic blankets may cause an alarm to be falsely sensitive. Most manufacturers recommend the use of cotton sheets and blankets.

- Make sure the alarm sound unit is positioned properly. Most wearable alarm manufacturers recommend their alarm be positioned high on your child's shoulder. Not only is it close to his ear in this position, it moves with him as he rolls in bed and it isn't muffled by blankets. Pad-type alarms have a sound unit that can be placed on a bedside table. Some can be moved far enough from the bed that your child must get up to turn it off. One type of alarm is positioned on the wrist. Make sure the cord is threaded under the pajama top and out the sleeve to prevent entanglement.

- If your child is taking sedating medication, is it possible to administer it at a different time of the day? Even cough, cold and allergy medications can interfere with your child's ability to respond to the alarm and stay dry.

- Ensure your child isn't pulling, rubbing or chewing the sensor cord. Try threading the cord up the back of the shirt to prevent this.

Avoid common parental mistakes

When a child wets the bed, parents take it personally. They ask, "What am I doing wrong?" When treating bedwetting, even the best intentioned parents can make common mistakes.

The most common mistake that parents make is giving up too soon: expecting results in the first few nights or getting discouraged that their child did not jump out of bed and run to the bathroom by himself. Remember, initially the alarm is for *you* to hear. Your child will respond to it later. Many parents give up prematurely because their child does not "hear" the alarm. Again, patience and time are of utmost importance.

Another common mistake is not using an effective alarm. In order to be effective, your child must be willing to use it every night. Comfort and "kid-appeal" are important. Large pads that fit into the underwear or vibratory alarms the size of a deck of cards are not comfortable; many children refuse to use them. The alarm must stay connected all night in order to be effective. Alarms with metal snap-type closures or hooks become disconnected easily, especially as the snaps and hooks bend with use. Both you and your child will be frustrated when he wakes up in the morning to a disconnected alarm and a wet bed. Children do not maliciously disconnect the alarm during the night, but reaching down to turn off the annoying noise is often their bodies' first response. Therefore, alarms with a two-step turn off and comfortable, secure attachments are preferred. (The Malem alarms have a unique two-step turnoff, requiring your child to do two sequential steps—remove the sensor from his underwear, then push a button on his shoulder.)

Another mistake parents make is thinking that if they tried an alarm in the past and their child did not get to dryness, it will never work for them. Many families find that retrying an alarm one or two years later provides very different results. Trying a different type of alarm often facilitates success.

Lastly, some times in a family's life are more optimal than others for using an alarm. Times of increased family stress, such as birth of new siblings, moving, job changes, vacations, etc., may not be ideal for the amount of effort required to be successful with a bedwetting alarm. If the program must be curtailed because of other family obligations, all is not lost. Often, the children can quickly relearn and get back on track after a few month hiatus.

Know when to stop

Knowing when to stop using the alarm is crucial to whether your child's dryness is permanent. Often, children become impatient and wish to discontinue use after four or five dry nights. Their wishful thinking convinces them that they no longer have bedwetting and don't need to use their alarms. Even as you document your child's progress, you must be sure he is truly dry before he stops using the alarm. Understand that if you stop using the alarm too early, chances are your child will start wetting again.

> *Before you stop using the alarm, your child should have 14 consecutive nights of dryness with nightly alarm use, and 14 additional dry nights using the alarm every other night.*

Frequent practice of a new response, called "over learning," is important in behavioral conditioning. That means even if your child seems to be dry, make sure by challenging his response. Before you discontinue alarm use, your child must have at least 14 *consecutive* dry nights, a few of them *fluid challenge nights.* If your child wets at all—on day two or day 13—you must start the counting over.

Conduct a fluid challenge

A fluid challenge is a technique in which your child drinks extra fluid in the evening. He then wears his alarm with the assurance he'll wake up when he needs to urinate, or he'll hold the urine until morning. Having the extra fluid on board challenges your child's apparent ability to wake up at his bladder's signal it is full and to empty it in the toilet. He wears the alarm just in case he needs a reminder. If your child wets on a challenge night, that indicates he should use the alarm longer.

It's a good strategy to conduct a fluid challenge on a weekend. More than two nights in a row can be exhausting. Remember, on a regular

Brian is 6, and he can't believe he has been dry for the last five nights. That bedwetting alarm must be doing its job! Five dry nights in a row is the longest run he has had in his whole life. He tells his parents he doesn't want to use his alarm any longer because he is cured. They want to believe him, but should they let him stop using the alarm so soon?

night it is appropriate for your child to drink enough fluid to quench his thirst. Do not routinely encourage fluids or severely limit them.

Wean your child off the alarm

Once your child achieves 14 dry nights in a row, some of them fluid challenge nights, have him begin to wear the alarm every other night until he again achieves 14 more consecutive dry nights. During this weaning period, children typically do very well. Only the occasional child will consistently wet on nights the alarm isn't in place. Again, if your child wets, he should use the alarm a few weeks longer, until you are certain he has internalized the new response and isn't dependent on having the alarm attached to him at night.

Remember, it takes children an average 12 weeks to become consistently dry. Many children have little setbacks along the way. Be patient and stick with it. Your child will love you for helping him become dry at night.

Children who relapse

Children who use alarms relapse much less frequently than children using any other method of bedwetting treatment. However, some children who have been dry for weeks or months will start wetting again. You can ignore an isolated wet night. In some situations, wetting can almost be expected. For example, if your child went to an evening sports activity, drank a large soda, fell asleep on the way home and didn't urinate before bed, you can expect a wetting accident. The next night should be a regular dry night.

If, however, there are two nights of wetness in one week without a change in routine, fluid intake or level of fatigue, you should resume using the alarm. Often, hearing and responding to the alarm for just one or two nights will get your child back on the path to dryness.

Don't wait for your child to start wetting every night again before resuming the alarm. By resuming the alarm after only two nights of wetness in one week, your child will quickly achieve the correct response. Again, have him wear the alarm until he has 14 consecutive nights of dryness.

Any illness, even colds or flu, can cause a temporary increase in wetting. Once your child begins to feel better, the wetting usually resolves. If your child seems completely well, but the wetting persists, resume using the alarm.

If you have to resume using the alarm, remind your child it is not a punishment but rather a gentle reminder to his brain what the correct response is. If your child has been dry for more than six months, then resumes wetting regularly and does not respond to the alarm, a visit to your health-care provider is warranted. Any new health condition, such as infection, diabetes, constipation, etc. should be ruled out for the cause of his secondary enuresis. You can find more information about secondary enuresis on page 23.

Part 2:
Beyond Seven Steps

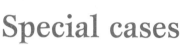

Special cases

Adolescents with bedwetting

There is no magic age at which bedwetting can no longer occur. Enuresis can persist into adolescence and can be particularly difficult to treat in this age group. Certainly, your child should have a complete physical examination and urologic evaluation by this time to rule out associated medical conditions. In most cases, these tests will be normal.

As many as 80 percent of adolescents with bedwetting have other relatives who wet the bed as well. In families who wait patiently for their child to stop bedwetting, up to 40 percent of teens have received no therapy for their bedwetting.[1] By the teen years, bedwetting has impacted their social development, limiting opportunities for sleepovers, camps, school trips, etc.

Teenagers can get to dryness.

As feelings of frustration and helplessness build, compliance and self-esteem decrease. Often, embarrassment and the feelings of being alone with this problem prevent the teen and parents from seeking medical intervention. Feelings that alarms and medications are only useful for younger children leave teens wondering if there is anything at all that they can do.

Teens can use alarms, too

Because parents don't have as much control over teens as younger children, you may have a more difficult time ensuring your teen's compliance with his bedwetting alarm. It's entirely his choice to hook up the alarm. That means he must be motivated and believe that using the alarm will end his bedwetting for the alarm to be effective. Stopping bedwetting in this age group is a very gradual but equally rewarding process.

You can increase compliance by helping your teen select the right alarm. Several manufacturers, such as Malem, provide solutions for people who are taller than six feet. The sensor cords are long enough to attach to the shoulder without difficulty. A comfortable, compact alarm such as the Malem ULTIMATE is well suited for an adolescent. This alarm has a sound and vibrating alert. As they progress, many teens like the confidentiality of the vibrate mode, which allows them to respond to the alarm independently.

Many teens like to wear baggy "boxer-type" underwear to bed. Remind your teen that alarms work best when attached to close-fitting briefs. The sooner the alarm can detect the first drop of moisture, the sooner it can sound to wake him. The alarm's sound also helps your child stop urination quickly, resulting in smaller spots in the bed and more urine left for the toilet. (Tip: Think about stopping your stream of urine during the daytime. It's much easier to stop early in the flow than after much of the bladder has already been emptied.) Your child can always wear the baggy boxers or pajama bottoms over close-fitting underwear with the alarm attached.

Another suggestion for teen-aged boys is to look down at their genitals when they get ready for bed. The direction their penis is situated will determine where the first drop of urine will come out. Placing the alarm sensor on the outside of their underwear in this area will facilitate the rapid sounding of the alarm.

> *Teens still need their parents' help to develop the proper response to the alarm.*

Adolescents can be independent in attaching the alarm to their underwear, double voiding before bed, taking medications and limiting after dinner fluids to water. That said, your child may continue to need your assistance to develop the proper response to the alarm. Because of your adolescent's physical size, he will have to get out of bed and walk to the bathroom by himself. Your role is that of verbally reminding him what to do, "That's your alarm. Get out of bed and walk to the bathroom."

If this gets no response, help him sit up and swing his legs over the side of his bed. Do not give up! He should walk to the bathroom, even if he says he does not need to urinate. Remind him to change into clean underwear and reattach the alarm. (Because of their increased bladder capacity, many adolescents wet only once a night. After the first two weeks of alarm use, if you have determined that your teen only urinates once per night, he doesn't need to reattach the alarm.)

Combination therapy for teens

A combination therapy of DDAVP, the drug that decreases total urine production, and a bedwetting alarm can be beneficial for teens. The adolescent takes a small amount of the medication at bedtime on nights spent in his own bed—a smaller dose than he needs to stay dry all night—and wears the alarm. Like younger children, he will most likely have wetting episodes later and later at night, eventually learning to stop his urine stream and stay dry. Combination therapy is particularly useful for teens because they often have more social obligations than younger children. They can attend overnight camp or sleepovers, leave their alarms at home, and take a dosage of DDAVP that keeps them dry all night. When they return home, they decrease their dosage and return to using the alarm until they are dry for 14 consecutive nights without medication.

Again, DDAVP doesn't maintain dryness for everyone. Teens who do stay dry with DDAVP have an easier time sleeping away from home. Teens who don't respond to DDAVP can use other dryness techniques when sleeping away from home, including double voiding, watching the type and quantity of fluid intake, using their own sleeping bags with waterproof liners and choosing the sleepover situations carefully.

Medications for other health problems

It is important for your teen to note any medications that he takes for other health conditions. The time of dosing and type of medication can adversely affect wetting. Medications taken for depression, anxiety, attention problems or even allergies can cause an increase in wetting. The exact mechanism for this is unknown. It may have to do with a change in the normal sleep patterns or an increase in thirst and/or urine production. In some teens, as their body adjusts to the medication, the wetting decreases. Dosing the medication earlier in the evening may help. (You should always contact your health-care provider before changing dosing times.)

Keeping records

Adolescents should keep their own personal progress records. They can see progress and count dry nights. They should record triggers, such as fatigue on Friday or Saturday nights, sleeping late on weekends, late-night sports events or increased soda intake. Once these triggers have been identified, paying particular attention to double voiding, alarm use and/or medication is beneficial. Getting out of bed to urinate early on a weekend morning when they intend to sleep late can prevent late morning accidents. Remind them that they can go back to bed!

Menstruation

Some female teens report that they wet more frequently around the time of their periods. One suggested theory is that cyclic fluid retention causes greater urine production as the body normalizes to premenstrual levels. For a female adolescent who is menstruating, using a bedwetting alarm can be a challenge. If she uses sanitary pads, she should place the pad in the usual position, the crotch of her panties, then attach the alarm's sensor in a different place on the outside of her panties. If she sleeps on her front, she should place the sensor in the front of the pad. If she sleeps on her back, she should place it behind the pad. While it may take a bit more urine to trigger the alarm, the alarm will still sense the moisture because it is not attached underneath the moisture-proof sanitary pad. If your daughter wears a tampon to sleep, she should attach her alarm as usual.

Alcohol and bedwetting

A mention should be made about ingesting alcohol and bedwetting. Because of increased evening fluid intake and the sedative effect of alcohol, incidence of bedwetting increases with alcohol intake. Your teen should be aware of this. Also, the use of DDAVP in conjunction with a large amount of oral fluids is not recommended. For these reasons, along with many other health concerns, drinking alcohol should be avoided.

Children with special needs

Children with special needs can also benefit from the use of bedwetting alarms. If your child has established daytime dryness, chances are she can also become dry at night.

If you have a child with special needs, it is important to understand your goal. Perhaps you simply want to be alerted when your child needs to be changed or helped to the toilet. In this case, a pad-type alarm, such as the Wet Call pad or Malem bedside, may be your best bet. Pad-type alarms sound when they detect moisture, but they don't require your child to attach any device to her clothing. Remember that your child should not wear disposable diapers or waterproof pants when using this type of alarm because the materials will prevent the alarm from sensing moisture. You could use a waterproof mattress overlay under the pad to decrease laundry.

An attachment for the Malem bedside alarm allows it to sound in your room in addition to or in place of sounding in your child's room. It also allows you to record any sound or voice as the alarm sound, which is essential if your child is sensitive to the loud single tone that alarms typically make. One family I know recorded their voices to remind their child to get up and go to the bathroom!

You might also consider using an alarm with disposable pants for your special needs child. You simply cut a small slit in the pants and insert the sensor. The Malem (standard sensor), WET-STOP and the DRI-Sleeper alarms can be used this way. The alarm units of these particular brands are designed to be attached to your child's shoulder to prevent detachment; be sure to run the sensor cord under her shirt. If your child has little movement during sleep, the alarm unit can also be attached to the bed.

If your goal is to teach your child how to wake to the need to urinate, make sure to choose a type of alarm that is acceptable to your child. Children with sensory problems might find a pad-type alarm to be acceptable. Children who are hearing impaired could use a Malem vibratory/auditory alarm. The vibration would alert them to go to the bathroom, and the sound would alert you to help your child. For hearing impaired parents, using a special infant monitor that lights in their room would help alert them. Children who are easily frightened by loud sounds can be acclimated by letting them "play" with the alarm for a day or two before using it. A recordable alarm allows you to record any familiar sound, music or a voice.

Children who wet only occasionally

Bedwetting alarms can also help children with intermittent wetting. Wetting a few nights a week can be as frustrating for children as wetting every night because the wet nights are usually unpredictable. Intermittent wetting still limits opportunities to spend nights with friends and still causes parent grief over increased laundry. Occasionally, parents believe their child has control over the wet or dry nights and is just "lazy." In reality, children have no idea what they did differently on wet or dry nights.

The bedwetting alarm should be placed and used in the manner described in Steps 5 and 6. Be sure to connect the alarm before bed each night, and that your child double voids. Kids who wet only occasionally become frustrated if they wear the alarm but stay dry all night, which makes compliance more difficult. You should also have your child drink an extra glass of fluid sometime between dinner and bedtime to increase the likelihood she will wet. While this seems a bit backwards, remember that you're trying to teach your child to respond to her full bladder by getting up and emptying it in the toilet. The extra fluid will give your child's brain more practice in recognizing the bladder's message and having the correct response. Remind her that practice makes perfect! As your child learns to wake herself with the use of the alarm or hold her urine until morning, even that extra fluid will not cause her to wet.

Once she is dry for 14 consecutive nights of using the alarm, then seven to 14 nights of using it every other night, she can stop using it. Since she will no longer wet, she can drink as much or as little as she wants in the evenings.

Siblings with bedwetting

Because bedwetting can be inherited, it often affects more than one child in the family. Again, it is not a "parenting defect," but genetically determined. As you recall, if one parent had bedwetting, 44 percent of his offspring will be similarly affected. If both parents have this history, 77 percent of their offspring will be affected.

It is not uncommon for siblings to have bedwetting.

Usually, the oldest sibling should be treated first. Once he becomes dry, his younger sibling could use the bedwetting alarm. (Some alarm systems have inexpensive replacement sensors, essentially providing the second child with a new alarm.)

Some families report that in bedwetting siblings who share a room, the younger child will wake up and go to the bathroom when the older child's alarm goes off. The younger sibling becomes dry simultaneously with the older one. Whether this is due to increased awareness, subconscious learning or just coincidence is unknown.

Some families prefer to treat siblings with bedwetting at the same time. They feel that since they are getting up at night anyway, they should finish with bedwetting all at once. If you choose to do this, have your children pick alarms that make different tones so you will know which child to respond to. (The different colored Malem alarms make different tones so that you can differentiate which child needs to get up.)

Remember when working with siblings that each child's response is unique. One child may alert to the alarm and progress quickly, while the other may require more parental assistance and persistence. This can be problematic when the younger child progresses more quickly than her older sibling. While a little sibling competition can encourage children to hook up and respond to their alarms, remind your children that each person's response is unique and cannot be compared to the other.

Children with daytime urgency/wetting

Before attempting treatment of nighttime wetting, your child should be reliably dry during the day. A few children with bedwetting also have symptoms of daytime leaking, urgency or frequency of urination. Wetting during the day is referred to as *diurnal enuresis,* and it is defined as wetting that is not caused by structural or neurologic factors in a child who is at least 5 years old.[2]

Daytime wetting problems past age 5 should be brought to the attention of your child's health-care provider. Testing may be recommended to rule out urinary tract problems. Wetting caused by urinary tract problems is referred to as incontinence and may require correction.

Daytime wetting where no urinary abnormalities are present often responds well to a timed voiding program. In some children, either the messages to void come very urgently or the messages are ignored until the bladder is completely full. Either way, your child may leak in his underwear or completely empty his bladder. To counter these responses, your child should void at scheduled times throughout the day, even if he doesn't feel the urge to do so at that time. A vibratory wrist watch, such as the VibraLITE 3 or MeDose, can be set to vibrate at approximately two-hour intervals. The vibration is a discreet reminder that only your child need know about. Prior arrangements can be made with his teacher to allow him to follow the watch's "direction" and go to the bathroom immediately when the watch reminds him to do so. Most teachers are very cooperative with this and want to assist your child in staying dry. Vibratory wrist watches are not easy to find in general stores; however the Bedwetting Store carries a full line. A small vibratory pager-like device, worn on the waistband or in the pocket, can also be set as a reminder to use the bathroom.

When setting the watch intervals, pay attention to your child's school schedule. Setting a vibration time when he cannot follow through is unreasonable. For example, if the watch vibrates at 4 p.m. but your child is on the bus at that time, he is unable to go to the toilet. By the time he arrives home, he may forget to go to the bathroom, and wetting occurs. A better scenario would be one in which the reminder occurred before loading the backpack and getting coats on at the end of the school day. Your child would start the trip home with an empty bladder, and no wetting would occur.

Your child's cooperation is a key factor in a timed voiding program. Most children would rather be dry than wet when given the choice. Initially, a reward or token for following the vibratory reminders for the entire day is appropriate. Only your child is aware of the discreet vibration when it happens. You don't need to remind him to use the toilet. If your child chooses to ignore the vibration on a regular basis, you should explore his motivation or attention-seeking behavior.

Because daytime wetting can be a source of frustration or conflict between parents and child, staying dry by using a timed voiding program can eliminate nagging or voiding reminders from parents. Many children learn to anticipate the vibration and begin to urinate independently when they sense the urge. The watch can be used just to tell time when this is established!

In addition to a timed voiding program, some children may benefit from the addition of the medication Ditropan. Your doctor or nurse practitioner can determine if this is right for your child and prescribe the correct dosage. This medication can help to make the bladder less "irritable" and send less urgent messages to the brain. As your child gets better at recognizing the messages, the medication can be decreased, and then discontinued, at your doctor's direction.

Sleepovers

The ability to stay all night with friends or grandparents or go to an all night camp is an important part of any child's social development. Some children want to do this as a 5-year-old, whereas others may be 9. Invitations for sleepovers often start by fourth grade. For children with bedwetting, these invitations can be a challenge. Anxious feelings about wetting in the presence of her friends may cause your child to make excuses and not attend their parties. You should make every effort for your child to attend without embarrassment.

Until your child becomes reliably dry, disposable pants are an easy sleepover solution. Work out a plan for when and where your child should put on her pants and how to dispose of them in the morning. Your child can discretely tuck the disposable pants into her overnight bag or sleeping bag. She can urinate one last time, then put on the pants in the bathroom or wiggle into them inside her sleeping bag if she's sleeping in one. Depending on your child's age and your relationship with the family, you can mention the arrangements to the adults. Be sure to ask them to keep this information confidential so as not to embarrass your child. You can give your child a plastic bag to put the pants in when she gets up in the morning. She can then put the bag in her overnight case and dispose of it when she gets home.

Disposable pants, medication and waterproof sleeping bag liners help children stay dry for sleepovers.

Waterproof sleeping bag liners are also useful products for children with intermittent or occasional wetting, or who have successfully used an alarm for some time but are not confident they can remain dry. These discreet liners will keep the outside of the sleeping bag and the carpet dry should she have a wet night. Liners are also helpful for extended camping trips. If your child has a wet night, simply remove the liner and replace it with a clean one. An added benefit: the liner keeps moisture from the ground from getting inside the sleeping bag.

Short-term medications such as DDAVP can also be useful for sleepovers. Since this medication works by decreasing the amount of urine produced that night, it often helps a child achieve dryness. You can find information about how to determine the correct dosage on page 32. For future events, you can give your child this dose for a single night, usually with great success.

Each child is different in his level of confidence in staying dry. Some children can be dry for two weeks and are willing to venture to a friend's house to spend the night. Other children may desire two months of dryness before they risk the embarrassment of an accident. There is no right or wrong response. Offering a safe environment, such as having a friend spend a night in your home initially or spending a night with an understanding relative, can help with the "jitters" of spending a night without bedding protection or medications. As your child builds confidence with this, they may be more willing to sleep at a friend's home.

References

[1] Nappo S, Del Gado R, Chiozza MI, Biraghi M, Ferrara P, Calone P. Nocturnal enuresis in the adolescent: a neglected problem. BJU Int. 2002; 90:92.

[2] Maizels M, Rosenbaum D, Keating B. Getting to Dry: How to Help Your Child Overcome Bedwetting. Boston. The Harvard Common Press; 1999.

Frequently asked questions

General bedwetting questions

1. How long does it take to reach complete dryness?

There are many elements that factor into bedwetting, but on average, dryness comes in 12 weeks.

2. Everyone tells me just to wait, that my son will "grow out of it." How do we know when to do something?

If your child is older than 6, is wetting every night, has a family history of wetting and expresses an interest in becoming dry, he is a good candidate for an alarm.

3. My child was slow in getting day toilet trained (4½ years). Is that why he is still wet at night? He is 6 now.

It is true that some maturation has to take place before daytime and nighttime dryness is achieved. In some children who have delays in getting dry during the day, it does take longer to get dry at night as well. You should see some progress in the next year. If not, using a bedwetting alarm when he is 7 or 8 would be appropriate intervention.

4. My son is 6 and wets every night. My husband told me that he also wet the bed until he was 12. He doesn't feel that we need to do anything special for our son because he'll eventually "outgrow" it. I feel bad for our son because I know he is becoming self-conscious about wetting and knows most of his friends don't wear disposable pants to bed. What do you recommend?

Based on your family history, your son probably faces many years of bedwetting unless intervention takes place. While it is fine to respond in a nonchalant and accepting manner, treatment would shorten the years of distress your son has to experience. After all, would you respond to your teenager with severe acne by saying, "You don't have to do any-thing, you'll outgrow it in five or 10 years." With current acne therapy available, no teen has to undergo the experience their parents may have gone through a generation ago. The same is true for bedwetting! With current bedwetting treatments, no child has to wait to "outgrow" it.

5. I am 33 years old, and I was a bedwetter until I was 13. My nephew has this problem as did my uncle. Is this inherited?

Yes, we know that there is a gene that controls for bedwetting and that it is an inherited condition. It makes some children feel better about them-selves to know that another family member also had this condition. Sharing your experiences and memories with your nephew may be helpful.

6. My child gets out of bed to urinate, but I hear him heading to the closet, the kitchen, or the hamper. Why does he do this?

It is not unusual that children with bedwetting will also be known to "sleepwalk." They are partially awakened by messages from the bladder but aren't fully awake to correctly respond. Making it difficult to urinate in places other than the bathroom can help. You could try putting a baby gate in the hall or blocking a closet or doorway. Putting a baby monitor in your room can alert you as to when your child is out of bed. Repeatedly guiding him to the proper location usually helps. Also, light-ing the bathroom with a nightlight can act as a beacon to draw him there. When your child's bedwetting alarm sounds, you should make sure that the toilet is his final destination.

7. I was told that the bedwetting alarm wakes the whole house, but not the bedwetting child.

This is probably the most misunderstood part of alarm usage. In fact, a child who is difficult to awaken is probably an excellent candidate for an alarm. The person who told you this most likely doesn't understand how alarms work.

8. My child is losing motivation and is discouraged after a few weeks of using the bedwetting alarm without any dry nights.

Keeping a log or calendar is a good way for your child to see that he is making progress. Even events like having small spots when your child awakens to the alarm or moving from wetting twice a night to only once is a sign of progress. Also, having the alarm sound five hours into the sleep cycle instead of two hours after your child has gone to bed is a sign of progress. Your child can be praised for any of these steps along the way to dryness. You can always refer to your calendar and show him that he is making progress while reminding him that patience is important.

9. What if I can't afford to lose a lot of sleep right now?

Some times are better in a family's life to begin a new treatment regimen. You might pick low stress times, such as summer or over school or work breaks. The first few weeks are the hardest. In the whole picture, though, your temporary lack of sleep will make a lifelong change for your child. Once your child begins to respond on her own, your role is much less important.

10. Why do children wet when they stop DDAVP?

The action of DDAVP is to decrease the quantity of urine produced that night. When the medication is stopped, the body resumes making a larger quantity of more dilute urine. If the bladder has grown to accommodate more urine or your child has learned to wake to messages from the bladder, he may have continued success in staying dry. In most cases, however, the wetting resumes when the medication is stopped.

11. My child is 11. He has taken DDAVP for four years, and it works great to keep him dry. If he misses one dose, though, he will wet that night. How many more years will he need this medicine?

It's hard to predict when your child will spontaneously stop wetting. This medicine does not provide permanent changes. It buys time until your child's body matures or until the family is ready to undertake a treatment approach using a bedwetting alarm. If he seems motivated, he could use the alarm when he is at home and the medication when he sleeps over. As he learns to wake to a full bladder, he will no longer require medication.

12. I have twins who both wet. How should I deal with this?
Each situation is different but if they both are wet most nights and are equally motivated to achieve dryness, you can purchase two bedwetting alarms that make different tones. If they share a room, you might temporarily move them to separate spaces. As you learn which child and alarm to respond to, and as they make progress, they can be moved back to the same room. Each child will progress at his own rate so avoid comparing progress.

13. I have three children. The two youngest ones have never wet at night. Their 10-year-old sister continues to wet. This is a source of sibling rivalry. What should we do?
Do not tolerate teasing or belittling of your bedwetting child by her siblings. You might explain that she has no control over her bedwetting, and she doesn't wet on purpose. Just as some children have difficulty learning to ride a bike or learning how to swim, some children have difficulty learning to stay dry at night. You can discretely assist your daughter in changing her bedding and underwear. If she does use a bedwetting alarm, you might let the siblings hear it and know that it is a noise that they need not respond to. You can explain that it is something that helps their sister learn to stay dry.

14. My son recently was very ill with strep throat. He resumed wetting even though he used the alarm successfully about six months ago and has not had an accident since then. What should I do?
Illness can cause bedwetting to reoccur. If he is completely well, has finished his medication, and continues to have wetting, you can resume the alarm. Discuss with your child that this is not a punishment but just a way of reminding his body what the proper response should be. Generally, when children need to resume using the bedwetting alarm,

the progress is much more rapid than it was in the beginning. Often, only a week or two of wearing the alarm will reestablish dryness.

15. My child was dry at night from ages 3 to 5. She started having nighttime accidents gradually, and now she wets every night. We've put her back in disposable pants. I have taken her to her pediatrician and there are no physical or urinary problems. There are no new stressors in her life. She has no problems during the day and has regular daily bowel movements. Now she is 7. What should we do?

Sometimes it is difficult to figure out why children have secondary enuresis (starts after a period of dryness). In some children, stressors such as parents' divorce, the birth of a sibling, changing schools or moving may coincide with wetting. Even after the stressor is no longer present, a child may continue to wet. If medical reasons have been ruled out, she will most likely respond to treatments used for children who have primary enuresis (have always wet). Using a bedwetting alarm to help her learn a new behavior is appropriate.

16. We had a salesperson come to our house offering bedwetting treatment for $2000. We want to do what is best for our child, but is this necessary?

Beware of companies that classify bedwetting as a sleep disorder and charge a lot of money to assist you with the use of a bedwetting alarm. While most children with bedwetting do have decreased arousal from sleep, so do many children who do not have bedwetting. Recent sleep studies done in controlled research settings have found that children can wet in any phase of the sleep cycle. Wetting does not occur only in the deep-sleep phase.

17. Recently, we have been waking our son up every two to three hours to go to the bathroom. It's getting old fast because none of us are getting any sleep. Do you have any suggestions?

What you are describing is very fatiguing for you. Picking an arbitrary time to wake him may keep him dry some nights but may be too late on other nights. Using a bedwetting alarm to pinpoint exactly when his bladder needs to empty is more effective and less tiring. Some nights, he may only need to urinate once and some nights more than that. The moisture sensor will only alert him and you when he actually needs to urinate.

18. I overheard my 8-year-old making an excuse as to why he didn't want to sleep at a friend's house. It seems that his bedwetting is beginning to affect his life. Is this a good time to intervene?

Yes, situations such as this are often opportune times for your child to be receptive to ways he can end bedwetting. Since learning to stay dry at night is a collaborative effort between child and parent, having the motivation to wear an alarm, double void, make dietary changes, etc. is half of the battle. By suggesting intervention at this time, your child will begin to feel that he has some control over his bedwetting, and his goal of staying at a friend's house can be achieved.

19. What if my child has friends over?

It could be a source of embarrassment if his friends hear an alarm go off. If it is early in the alarm training program, your child can resort to the use of a disposable pant for the night, and then resume the alarm when he returns to his regular schedule.

20. What can I do about sleepovers?

Several options are available, depending on the age and comfort level of your child. Discreet use of disposable pants is an easy option for a younger child. Provide a sealable plastic bag so she can bring it home to dispose of it. A waterproof sleeping bag liner would protect your child from having any leaking onto carpet or bedding if she went to a party where sleeping bags would be used. Use of medication such as DDAVP provides short-term dryness. (Remember that the correct dose should be determined in advance of the special event.)

21. My child has an important sleepover coming up. How much time should we allow for her to become predictably dry?

Obviously, if she wakes on her own to the alarm, progress will be faster. Some of the most difficult-to-arouse sleepers require a few weeks to

Seven Steps to Nighttime Dryness

even hear the alarm on their own. The average length of alarm conditioning is about three months. Many children like to be dry for a few weeks before they attempt a sleepover. If the important event is before they are dependably dry, follow the tips in question 20. Once she is home, she can resume the alarm.

22. My child is 12. Most of the time, he doesn't wet when staying with friends. Why is this?

Some children do not sleep as soundly or for as many hours when they spend the night outside their own home. Because of this, some can stay dry for one night. (The ability to do this is a huge advantage for your child). Over a few nights' time, however, fatigue from missing sleep or increased comfort in the new bed can make wetting resume. Remember that no child wants to wake up wet, and he certainly does not wet on purpose when he is at home.

23. I have a 13-year-old daughter with bedwetting. She did well over the summer but when school and sports started, she had more wetting. It seems that she is so tired that she just doesn't wake up. What should we do?

Fatigue definitely plays a part in the number of wet nights. Until her body permanently achieves the new response of waking, no matter how tired she is, using a bedwetting alarm as an external reminder is beneficial. Often, as the routine of the school year becomes established and her body becomes more conditioned for her sports, dryness will resume. Until that happens, have her use the alarm.

24. My son goes to his dad's house every other weekend. Bedwetting is not a problem there. Why does he wet only at my house?

This is similar to situations at sleepovers where children can maintain dryness. Maybe your son is a little less comfortable and sleeps lighter at dad's house. Also, the nighttime routine, bedtime and diet can be different. Maybe dad walks him to the bathroom when he gets up in the night. The main thing to remember is that your child is not wetting on purpose at your house. If you are using a bedwetting alarm at your house, enlisting the other parent's cooperation in the routine is helpful, especially in the initial phases.

25. Our 10-year-old son has ADD (Attention Deficit Disorder) and is on medication. We've noticed that he wets more frequently on weekends and during the summer when he isn't taking his medication. Is there any relationship here?

Bedwetting is a little more common in children with ADD than in the general population. The exact mechanism for this is not known. It does appear that when children can pay attention to the external messages that their body receives, they can also attend more easily to their body's internal messages.

General alarm questions

1. Aren't all alarms the same?

All alarms work by making a loud noise and/or vibration when they sense moisture. After that, you have choices. It's important to choose an alarm your child will use every night until he is dry. That means it must be visually appealing—think "kid cool"—comfortable, dependable and easy to use. Alarms can vary in the manner they attach to clothing; beware of metal snap closures because they can easily become detached if your child moves a lot in sleep. Alarms also differ in the way they alert your child. Some make a loud noise, others vibrate. Some vibrate and make a loud noise. Some alarms allow you to record a sound or voice you know your child will respond to. Keep in mind that children who are difficult to arouse usually require a loud sound to wake them and their parents; for this reason a vibratory-only alarm is not recommended for your child.

2. What is the difference between a one-tone alarm and a multiple-tone alarm?

With a one-tone alarm, each time the sensor detects moisture you will hear the same alarm sound. With multiple-tone alarms, you will hear a different sound each time the alarm turns on. For example, with the eight-tone Malem alarm, the first night it goes off, you will hear one

Seven Steps to Nighttime Dryness

sound. The next time it goes off, either that same night or the next night, you will hear a different sound. Choosing a one-tone or multiple-tone alarm is your own personal preference. There is no research to indicate that one is more effective than the other.

3. How loud are the alarms?

Most alarms are 80 to 90 decibels, as measured from the position on your child's shoulder. This is not loud enough to contribute to hearing loss but loud enough for parents in a nearby bedroom to hear. The average sleeping adult would respond to noises in the 40 to 45 decibel range.

4. How long does the alarm sound for?

The sound remains on as long as it senses moisture and/or the alarm is reset.

5. How successful are bedwetting alarms?

Numerous studies have been done over the past 10 to 15 years to measure the effectiveness of moisture-sensing alarms. Results vary, but report 60 to 80 percent success with a low relapse rate.

6. What do I do when I hear the alarm turn on/sound (parents)?

Once you hear the alarm, you should go into your child's room, wake her up and assist her to her feet. The alarm can be disconnected and turned off when she is standing.

7. But hasn't my son already wet by the time the alarm sounds? Isn't it "too late"?

Initially, your child will have completely emptied his bladder by the time you get to him. Everyone starts this way. Over time, he will release smaller amounts of urine before he or you responds to the alarm.

8. Will the alarm "shock" my child?

No. Alarms are not designed to shock anyone, but rather sense moisture and sound an alarm.

9. What happens if my alarm won't shut off?

If the alarm continues to sound, in most cases it is still sensing moisture. Drying the sensor or pad thoroughly before reattaching is important. Also, since urine residue can build up on the sensor over time, it is helpful to clean it with warm, soapy water on a regular basis.

10. My child can sleep through anything, even his alarm clock. Will my child hear the alarm?

Bedwetting alarms are not likely to awaken a bedwetting child initially. Children initially need assistance in awakening to the alarm. This is why it is so important to have an audible alarm to alert someone else in the household to assist your child. Achieving nighttime dryness is a GRADUAL learning process that requires parental participation.

11. What if our house is situated so that we (parents) can't hear the alarm?

Some parents use an infant monitor in their room so they can hear the bedwetting alarm sound in their child's room and help them respond to it.

12. I'm worried that the alarm will wake up everyone in my household. What can we do to prevent this?

Explain to the siblings that everyone in the family has things they need to learn. This child needs help in learning to stay dry at night, and the alarm helps him learn this. Allow the siblings to hear what the alarm sounds like, and instruct them to go back to sleep if they hear this during the night. Generally, the alarm's sound is not a problem for other members of the household. Occasionally, mom and dad may have a little difficulty getting back to sleep, however. You may want to take turns responding to the alarm with your child so that you don't become overly tired.

13. My child is disoriented when I wake him when I go to bed. Why will the alarm be any different?

The alarm sounds at the precise time that your child needs to urinate—not 15 minutes earlier or 15 minutes later. Even though your child may be disoriented in the early hours after going to sleep, you will begin to see that she is more easily aroused as her body begins to associate the feeling of a full bladder with waking and walking to the bathroom.

14. My child doesn't even remember getting up at night when the alarm goes off. How can she learn?

Subconscious learning takes place. Some children become dry without remembering the actual process of hearing the alarm.

15. Will my child be too tired to go to school the next day?

Children are very resilient. Even if the alarm goes off more than once a night, they have the ability to go back to sleep immediately and often not remember much of it in the morning. Parents, however, may feel very tired the next day. It often takes adults a little longer to fall back asleep, depending on the point in their sleep cycle that they awoke. Remember that the first month is the most difficult. It typically gets easier from there on.

16. Can my child wear disposable pants when using the alarm?

In most cases, you shouldn't use an alarm with disposable pants. First, the highly absorbent materials can easily "wick away" moisture when your child wets and prevent the alarm from sounding appropriately. The result is a missed learning opportunity and the potential for mistakenly thinking that your child was dry. Secondly, it is very difficult to monitor progress, especially as your child reduces the amount he wets. Most alarms were designed to be used with cloth underwear.

17. I wake my child and take him to the bathroom before I go to bed. Should I continue to do this when we use the alarm?

No, let the alarm do the waking for you. That way, your child will learn to associate a full bladder with going to the toilet.

18. How long does my child have to wear the alarm?

When used properly, the average time to achieve dryness is about 12 weeks. Some children take less time and some take months more. Once a child has 14 consecutive dry nights, you can have them wear the alarm every other night for 14 more nights. If they are still dry, you can stop the alarm at that point. This period of "over learning" keeps you from stopping the process prematurely and assures that your child has learned the proper response.

19. We have used the alarm for a whole week and our child is not dry yet. Should we assume the alarm won't work for our child?

Absolutely not. Establishing a new behavior through the use of a bed-wetting alarm is a gradual process that takes time. Using the alarm for this short time and expecting dryness is unrealistic. Remember that the average child takes 10 to 12 weeks to get to dryness. The first month is the hardest, and then you will begin to see results.

20. I read that the average child takes about 12 weeks to become dry using an alarm. My child has used it for 12 weeks now. He no longer wets every night, just once or twice a week. He only has small spots on his underwear that trigger the alarm on his wet nights. How much longer will we need to use the alarm?

He certainly is progressing in the right direction. Since each child's rate of response is different, continue to use the alarm until he reaches 14 consecutive dry nights. Step 7 discusses how to know when your child is ready to stop using the alarm.

21. How do I tell that my child is doing well/progressing/responding to the alarm?

Your child begins to wake up to the alarm before the parent; the wet spot on your child's pajamas or bed begins to become smaller; the wetting episode occurs later into the night rather than soon after your child has gone to bed. These are all signs of progress.

22. My child is dry about half of the time now and doesn't want to wear the alarm every night.

Intermittent wetting can be frustrating. Remind her that she should wear the alarm every night until 14 consecutive dry nights are achieved. If she wears the alarm only on the nights she "feels like it," she will miss valuable nights of learning—the rare nights that she wets and the alarm sounds. Ultimately, it will take longer for her to become consistently dry if she wears the alarm only sporadically.

23. Our son is 9. He wets every night. I once bought an alarm when he was 6, but the loud noise upset him and he refused to try it. He is strong-willed and I decided to back off. What course of action do you recommend?

Now that he is older, you may be able to present how an alarm works a little differently to enlist his cooperation. Children of his age are often quite motivated to do what it takes to become dry. Remind him that this is just a noise to help him learn when to get up to go to the bathroom. It can not hurt him in any way. Having him practice turning the alarm on and off in the daytime will help him get used to that particular sound. Things that frighten a 6-year-old are much different than those that frighten a 9-year-old.

24. Why is it a good idea to wear an alarm unit attached to the shoulder?

By placing the alarm close to the ear, you maximize the chances of your child hearing and waking up to the alarm. Your child can easily move from front to back (and vice versa) and the alarm will remain in the correct position without being in the way. Also, the sound is less likely to be muffled by blankets and pillows with a shoulder rather than a wrist or waist alarm.

25. My child moves around a lot in his sleep. Will the alarm stay put?

Most alarms will stay attached with sleep movement. Most manufacturers recommend running the cord up the inside of your child's T-shirt or pajama top so it won't be inadvertently pulled on or become entangled as your child sleeps.

26. My son seems to disconnect the alarm in his sleep, then rolls back over and goes back to sleep before I hear it. What can I do?

You may need to double secure the alarm by placing a safety pin or piece of adhesive tape about an inch up on the cord. Your child would have to be a little more awake to unfasten these things and should be able to get to the bathroom. (You might suspect this is happening if your child wakes up wet in the morning with an alarm on the floor or disconnected.) Some alarms, such as the Malem one, have a two-step process to shut them off to keep this from happening.

27. My child used an alarm that vibrated and fit into her underwear. I would walk into her room in the morning and find the alarm on the floor and her bed soaked. She didn't get up to go to the bathroom and doesn't remember disconnecting the alarm. Does this experience mean that she won't be successful with any type of alarm?

Alarms that provide vibration only do not allow for assistance from the parents. A few children respond to vibration only, but the majority need noise so that their parents can be alerted and remind them of the appropriate response. Disconnecting the alarm and rolling back over to go to sleep was the wrong response and would not help your daughter become dry.

28. What if my child won't wear the alarm?

Allow your child to turn the alarm off and on during their waking hours. Assure her that it's only a noise—that it can't hurt her. Remind her that this is a kind of "gadget" that will help her learn a new response to a full bladder, to wake up and go to the bathroom instead of wetting. There are pad types of alarms that your child can lay on if she refuses to have a sensor connected to her underwear.

29. What if my child is afraid of the alarm?

Have your child practice with the alarm at least three times before he goes to bed the first night. This will help him to become familiar with the alarm's tones and/or vibration. It also helps mom and dad become familiar with the tones so they don't wake up thinking the bedwetting alarm is the smoke detector or burglar alarm.

30. My daughter says the alarm is not comfortable. What type is best?

Especially with young girls, I recommend smaller alarms that can easily be attached to the outside of the crotch of the panties. Some girls wear a pair of soft, loosely fitting underwear or pajama bottoms over the top of the panties with the alarm attached, to sandwich the sensor in place.

31. My child is very sensitive to touch and refuses to use a wearable alarm. What other options are there?

There are many different makes and models of bedwetting alarms available. Your child may do well with a moisture-sensing pad-type of alarm. This is placed in a pillowcase or under a towel beneath your child. It senses urine and makes a loud sound, alerting child and parents that they need to get up. There are no cords or sensors for your child to wear with this type of device. Another type of wireless alarm consists of snapping a small transmitter to the outside of specially designed underwear. It transmits the signal to a wall unit to alert child and parent that they need to get up.

32. Can medications and an alarm be used together?

Yes. The purpose of using an alarm is to learn a new behavior. Medications, such as DDAVP or Ditropan, can be used with an alarm to help a child achieve dryness. These medications decrease urine production and allow the bladder to hold more at a time. As your child gets to dryness, the medications are gradually discontinued. The new behavior remains and is a permanent response. Combining medication and alarms in children who have used each independently will often help them achieve success. This is discussed on page 35.

33. My child has been on numerous medicines over the years and used an alarm a few years ago, yet he still wets. Is there anything we can do?

Treating bedwetting can be very frustrating. Often combining treatments or retrying an alarm when a child is older can stop the wetting. If it has been several years since an alarm was used, you may be surprised at your child's response now that he is older. Make sure that the alarm that you choose is not easily disconnected, is comfortable and durable and makes sound. Remember that sound is necessary initially so you can be alerted that your child needs to get up.

34. How should my teen-aged daughter attach the alarm when she is menstruating?

If she wears a sanitary napkin in her underwear, the alarm sensor should be placed in front or back of the waterproof area. The best placement will depend on her usual sleeping position: back-sleepers should place the sensor behind the napkin, and front-sleepers should place it in front of the napkin.

35. Does insurance pay for the alarm?

It depends on your own policy and whether your insurance company considers it a covered benefit. Bedwetting alarms can be classified as durable medical equipment (DME). Your insurance company may assign a different local code. The only way to be certain is to contact your carrier. Even if the alarm is not a covered benefit, it is a relatively inexpensive way to help your bedwetting child.

36. Can I use an alarm for daytime wetting as well?

Vibratory watches are recommended for daytime wetting/voiding. A timed voiding program, where your child is reminded to urinate at regular intervals of time is very helpful. The vibration discreetly reminds your child to use the bathroom. They are typically set for about two hour intervals. Children with sensory deficits or developmental delays can use alarms during the day to alert their caretaker and themselves that wetting is occurring. Over time, the association of the sound and a full bladder takes place.

Helpful cleaning tips

1. How do I minimize wet sheets I have to wash?

Before beginning a treatment program, using disposable pants is acceptable. Once you start using an alarm, your child should be in cloth underwear. To help with this transition, many parents use washable, waterproof mattress overlays. These are quilted, absorbent pads that lie on top of the sheets. Your child begins the night laying on one of these, then changes to a clean one when he wets. Pads with tuck-in sides to help with placement are available for children who move a lot in their sleep.

Children with bedwetting may also get their blankets and comforters wet (depending on their position when they wet or how twisted up in the bedding they are). Using easily laundered, thinner blankets and bedspreads are preferable to bulky bedding.

2. How can I remove urine odor from the bathroom?

Because urine can seep into the tile grout or wood in a bathroom, it is sometimes difficult to clean completely. An enzyme-based product like Urine-Erase™ will remove stubborn urine stains from places like the bathroom.

3. How can I remove urine stains from the mattress?

Using an enzyme based product like Urine-Erase™ is the most effective way to clean a mattress. Once the mattress is clean, using a zippered vinyl cover will protect it from further stains until your child is reliably dry. The Resources section at the end of this book contains information about purchasing this item.

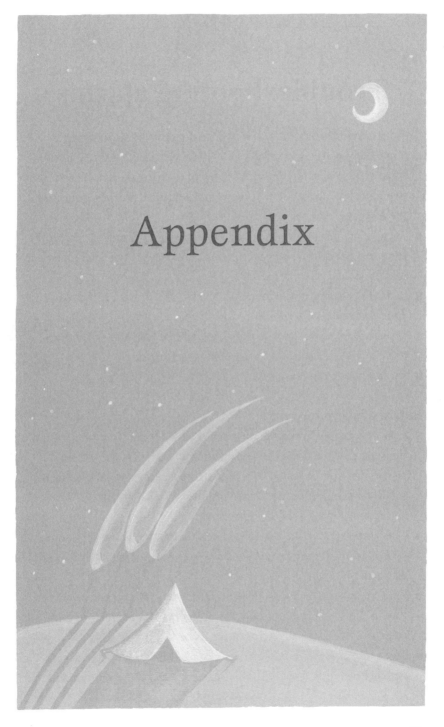

Appendix

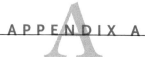

Troubleshooting alarms

Children switching the alarm off and going back to sleep

■ Some body-worn alarms are easily disconnected from the underwear. Strategic use of safety pins, duct tape or layering the sensor between two pairs of underwear will increase the difficulty of disconnecting the alarm.

■ The Malem alarm should not be switched off by removing the cord from the alarm unit. Insist that your child use the two step process to turn it off.

■ Move the alarm unit further from the bed for the bed mats, requiring your child to get out of bed to turn it off.

■ Use a baby monitor in your room so you can hear the alarm sound more quickly. Ensure that your child is getting up.

■ Re-emphasize the reason why you are using the alarm.

Failure of alarm to sound

■ Test the alarm. On wearable models, complete the circuit by closing the sensor or touching the sensor with moisture (Note: Malem alarms can also be tested by removing the sensor cord and using a small metal object to touch the wire prongs inside the jack. The alarm unit should sound when doing this).

■ Check and replace the batteries. Even though the alarm may sound when testing, it may be less sensitive if batteries are not sufficiently charged.

■ On some pad-type models, it is necessary to apply pressure and moisture at the same time in order to test the mat. The moisture must cross two of the sensor strips at the same time.

■ The sensor may be less sensitive because it is coated with urine residue. Cleaning most wearable sensors with soapy water and an old toothbrush will renew the sensor. Pads should also be cleaned with soapy water regularly if you have a pad-type model.

- Check the connection between the sensor, cord and alarm unit.
- Make sure the wearable alarm is connected to the clothing properly and is reattached after the first wetting episode.
- Contact the manufacturer or major outlets for replacement parts.
- The alarm unit should not become wet. If this occurs, dry thoroughly and replace batteries.
- For wearable alarms, make sure the sensor is where the first drop of urine hits the underwear.
- For pad-type alarms, ensure that your child isn't rolling off it.

False alarms

- May be caused by perspiration. Reduce amount of bedding and room temperature.
- Make sure wearable alarms are located on outside of underwear.
- Do not place occlusive rubber pants or disposable diapers over the top of underwear. The sensor may get unduly saturated, continue to sense moisture and sound.
- Sensor needs to be cleaned. Stale urine coupled with fresh urine and/or perspiration will trigger the alarm.
- The underwear is too thin. Cotton underwear is better than nylon or polyester blend.
- Static electricity in the bedding can cause false alarms, especially in pad-type alarms. Use cotton bedding, not fluffy acrylic blankets.
- Placing a thick cotton towel or drawsheet over the pad-type alarms make them less sensitive to perspiration.
- Batteries may need to be replaced. Low power can cause erratic alarms.
- If the false alarms continue after trying these suggestions, it is possible the alarm isn't working properly. Contact the manufacturer for further tests.

Lack of progress

- Don't use the alarm intermittently. Learning takes longer with intermittent behavioral reinforcement.

- Use the alarm until the child is consistently dry. Stopping early may cause wetting to resume.
- Parents must participate regardless of their child's age. Your role is to ensure that your child gets out of bed as a response to the alarm.
- Changing type of alarm, for example, from body-worn to pad-type, or sound and vibration may help.
- Resuming use of the alarm after a few months break can help discouraged children.

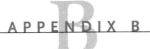

APPENDIX B

Resources for additional information

We've compiled a list of resources to help you research bedwetting, read more about the topic or purchase bedwetting products for your child.

Online

Visit www.bedwettinghandbook.com, the *Seven Steps to Nighttime Dryness* web site, for updated information and additional frequently asked questions. You will also find links to additional bedwetting web sites including where to purchase items for your child.

For a free mail order catalog of bedwetting products, contact the Bedwetting Store (800-214-9605) or visit their web site.

Bedwetting Store
BWS Catalogs
PO Box 337
Olney, MD 20830-0337
800-214-9605
www.bedwettingstore.com
catalogs@bedwettingstore.com

Enuresis Associates
Dorsey Hall Medical Center
9501 Old Annapolis Rd, Ste 201
Ellicott City, MD 21042
301-774-1349
www.dryatnight.com

Publications

Several books are currently in print that provide information ranging from comprehensive reviews on the evaluation and management of bedwetting to children's books geared toward younger readers to assure them that bedwetting is a common childhood condition.

Books for Parents

Getting to Dry: How to Help Your Child Overcome Bedwetting by Max Maizels MD, et al. January 1999

Getting to Dry is a comprehensive book about bedwetting. Intended for parents and health professionals, the experts at one of the country's leading centers for treating childhood wetting explain how parents can speed up the clock and children can wake up happy and dry. They cover the pros and cons of wetting alarms, drug therapies, and changes in diet and sleeping schedules. 272 pages.

Dry All Night: The Picture Book Technique That Stops Bedwetting by Alison Mack, David Wilensky. September 1990

Picture book technique that helps stop bedwetting. Part 1 provides parents with information about coping with bedwetting and Part 2 is an illustrated story for children. 174 pages.

No More Bedwetting : How to Help Your Child Stay Dry by Samuel J. Arnold, MD. December 1997

No More Bedwetting helps parents and caregivers understand what causes bedwetting and what can be done about it. Shows parents how to handle each type of bedwetting, whatever the cause. Discusses medical causes and interventions. 208 pages.

Books for Children

Dry Days, Wet Nights (A Concept Book) by Maribeth Boelts, Kathy Parkinson (Illustrator). September 1996

For children ages two to five. Little Bunny has given up his diapers because he can stay dry all day. At night, though, he wets the bed, since he can't seem to wake up enough to get to the bathroom.

Sammy the Elephant and Mr. Camel: A Story to Help Children Overcome Enuresis While Discovering Self-Appreciation by Joyce C. Mills, et al, Germaine Cook (Illustrator).
March 1989
For children ages four to eight. Sammy is a little elephant who can't hold his water in this delightful fable for helping children overcome bedwetting and to believe in their own self-worth.

Do Little Mermaids Wet Their Beds? by Jeanne Willis, Penelope Jossen (Illustrator). April 2001
For children ages four to eight. This book is about Cecelia, a clever girl with a problem that won't go away—bedwetting. Cecelia has a wonderful dream, about a mermaid who reveals that she, too, has had this difficulty.

Weekly progress chart

Completing the Weekly Progress Chart each morning is the easiest way to record accurate data. It is more difficult to reconstruct several nights of information if you don't do it on a daily basis. Recalling what happens from one night to the next is not easy!

Remember:

■ Getting a cooperation sticker requires a ✓ in all 3 behavior categories

■ A dry night sticker is awarded if your child sleeps all night dry or if they get up before the alarm sounds

■ If the alarm sounds more than once per night, record each time

■ Record the size of the spot to monitor progress
  S = the size of a baseball
  M = the size of a cantaloupe
  L = the size of a basketball or larger

■ Notes can include unusual activities, new foods or drinks, illness, medications, etc.

The importance of creating a visual reward system is discussed on page 53. Comparing the current weekly chart with previous charts will help your child see the progress they have made. You may reproduce this blank chart, or visit www.bedwettinghandbook.com to print a version.

Weekly progress chart

W E E K 1

Date	Wore Alarm	Double Voided	Nighttime Cooperation	Dry Night	Woke Before Alarm	Woke to Alarm	Time of Alarm	Size of Spot S—M—L	Notes/Contributing Factors
MON									
TUE									
WED									
THU									
FRI									
SAT									
SUN									

Weekly progress chart

W E E K 2

Date	Wore Alarm	Double Voided	Nighttime Cooperation	Dry Night	Woke Before Alarm	Woke to Alarm	Time of Alarm	Size of Spot S–M–L	Notes/Contributing Factors
MON									
TUE									
WED									
THU									
FRI									
SAT									
SUN									

Seven Steps to Nighttime Dryness

Weekly progress chart

Date	Wore Alarm	Double Voided	Nighttime Cooperation	Dry Night	Woke Before Alarm	Woke to Alarm	Time of Alarm	Size of Spot S–M–L	Notes/Contributing Factors
MON									
TUE									
WED									
THU									
FRI									
SAT									
SUN									

Weekly progress chart

W E E K 4

Date	Wore Alarm	Double Voided	Nighttime Cooperation	Dry Night	Woke Before Alarm	Woke to Alarm	Time of Alarm	Size of Spot S–M–L	Notes/Contributing Factors
MON									
TUE									
WED									
THU									
FRI									
SAT									
SUN									

Weekly progress chart

W E E K 5

Date	Wore Alarm	Double Voided	Nighttime Cooperation	Dry Night	Woke Before Alarm	Woke to Alarm	Time of Alarm	Size of Spot S—M—L	Notes/Contributing Factors
MON									
TUE									
WED									
THU									
FRI									
SAT									
SUN									

Weekly progress chart

Date	Wore Alarm	Double Voided	Nighttime Cooperation	Dry Night	Woke Before Alarm	Woke to Alarm	Time of Alarm	Size of Spot S–M–L	Notes/Contributing Factors
MON									
TUE									
WED									
THU									
FRI									
SAT									
SUN									

W E E K 7

Weekly progress chart

Date	Wore Alarm	Double Voided	Nighttime Cooperation	Dry Night	Woke Before Alarm	Woke to Alarm	Time of Alarm	Size of Spot S–M–L	Notes/Contributing Factors
MON									
TUE									
WED									
THU									
FRI									
SAT									
SUN									

Weekly progress chart

Date	Wore Alarm	Double Voided	Nighttime Cooperation	Dry Night	Woke Before Alarm	Woke to Alarm	Time of Alarm	Size of Spot S–M–L	Notes/Contributing Factors
MON									
TUE									
WED									
THU									
FRI									
SAT									
SUN									

Weekly progress chart

WEEK 9

Date	Wore Alarm	Double Voided	Nighttime Cooperation	Dry Night	Woke Before Alarm	Woke to Alarm	Time of Alarm	Size of Spot S–M–L	Notes/Contributing Factors
MON									
TUE									
WED									
THU									
FRI									
SAT									
SUN									

Appendix C—Weekly progress chart

Weekly progress chart

Date	Wore Alarm	Double Voided	Nighttime Cooperation	Dry Night	Woke Before Alarm	Woke to Alarm	Time of Alarm	Size of Spot S–M–L	Notes/Contributing Factors
MON									
TUE									
WED									
THU									
FRI									
SAT									
SUN									

Seven Steps to Nighttime Dryness

Weekly progress chart

W E E K ___

Date	Wore Alarm	Double Voided	Nighttime Cooperation	Dry Night	Woke Before Alarm	Woke to Alarm	Time of Alarm	Size of Spot S–M–L	Notes/Contributing Factors
MON									
TUE									
WED									
THU									
FRI									
SAT									
SUN									

GLOSSARY

Anti-diuretic hormone (ADH)
also known as vasopressin; hormone secreted by the pituitary gland that regulates the excretion of urine by the kidney.

Bladder
small muscular balloon that stores urine.

Constipation
hard, dry or infrequent bowel movements.

Desmopressin
a synthetic hormone used to supplement naturally secreted vasopressin; reduces the amount of urine produced by the kidney; also know by trademark DDAVP.

Diurnal enuresis
wetting that occurs in the daytime while awake.

Encopresis
soiling of bowel movement in the underwear by a child who is over 4 years old.

Enuresis
an involuntary discharge of urine not due to structural urologic factors; wetting. Can be further defined as diurnal, nocturnal, primary or secondary.

Frequency
how often urination occurs; increased frequency may occur with small bladder capacity or urinary infections; average person urinates five to nine times per day.

Functional bladder capacity
the amount of urine the bladder holds when it alerts the brain that it is full.

Hormone
a substance produced by an organ that travels by the bloodstream to act upon a distant tissue.

Kidney
a paired organ in the body that produces urine.

Lifting
a technique where the child is awakened or carried to the bathroom to urinate.

Nocturnal enuresis
wetting that occurs during sleep.

Oxybutynin
a medication that allows bladder muscles to relax and hold more urine; also known by trademark Ditropan.

Pelvic floor muscles
groin muscles that help to control the flow of urine.

Primary enuresis
wetting that has always been present (primary nocturnal enuresis is wetting that has always been present during sleep).

Relapse
two or more wet nights in a week after a prolonged period of dryness.

Secondary enuresis
wetting that occurs after at least six months of consistent dryness.

Serotonin
a substance that regulates cyclic body processes such as sleep and memory.

Timed voiding
emptying bladder during the day at regular intervals of time (e.g., every two hours).

Timed voiding program
technique using a device such as a watch or timer to vibrate or sound as a reminder to urinate.

Tryptophan
an amino acid formed from protein during digestion, triggers serotonin release.

Urgency
the sensation of the need to urinate very soon.

Ureter
small tube that carries urine from the kidney to the bladder.

Urethra
tube that carries urine from the bladder to the outside of the body.

Urinary system
responsible for producing urine, storing it and getting rid of it.

Urinary tract infection (UTI)
a condition where bacteria (germs) grow anywhere along the tracts where the urine passes, causing an infection. Can occur in the kidney, ureter, bladder or urethra.

Vasopressin
see anti-diuretic hormone (ADH).

Voiding
the act of excreting urine.

Siblings
  reactions, 17, 90
  rivalry, 84
  treatment of, 76, 84
  with bedwetting, 76
Sleep
  apnea, 23
  decreased arousal from, 11–12, 16, 29, 85, 90
Sleep walking, 49, 82
Sleeping arrangements, using alarm, 49
Sleeping bag, liners, 27, 79
Sleepovers
  and bedwetting, 78, 86–87
  use of medication for, 29, 86
Special needs children
  goals, 74
  use of bedwetting alarm, 74–75
Supportive
  lifting, 28
  restricting fluids, 27
  treatments, 21
  waiting, 26

Teens
  combination therapy for, 72
  keeping records, 73
  parental assistance with, 71–72
  use of alarms, 70
  with bedwetting, 18, 62, 87
Timed voiding program
  for daytime wetting, 76–78
  use of vibratory watch in, 77
Treatment of bedwetting, starting, 20–21

Urinary
  control, development of, 7–8
  disorders, 16, 22
  infections, 15, 22
  system, 6–8
Urine stains, removal, 96

Waterproof bedding
  disposable pads, 27
  sleeping bag liners, 27
  washable pads, 27, 51–52
Wearable alarms
  comparison, 45
  description, 39
Wireless alarms, 41